Healthyism

Healthy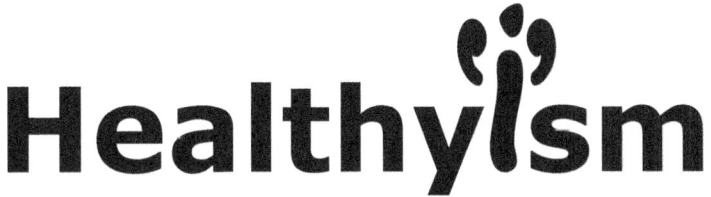sm

Healthy I, Healthy World!

The Evolutionary Practice of Constructive Consciousness

OR

How to Improve Your Life

AND Save Our World

Gary Drisdelle

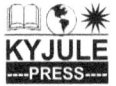

Copyright © 2010 by Gary J. Drisdelle

Published by
KYJULE PRESS

All rights reserved. No part of this publication may be reproduced, stored in a retrieval system, or transmitted in any form or by any means, electronic, mechanical, photocopying, recording, or otherwise – except by a reviewer who may quote brief passages in a review – without prior written permission from the author.

Editorial and Creative Contributions: Renne La Tulippe, Ricky Anderson, Jason Maloney and Lisa Corcoran
Book and Cover Design: Corcoran & Nelli, LLC
Author Photography: Monica Jones

Books are available at substantial discounts when used to support others in *practicing constructive consciousness.* For additional copies and discount information visit the HealthyIsm website at:

www.HealthyIsm.com

Library and Archives Canada Cataloguing in Publication

Drisdelle, Gary , 1961-
   HealthyIsm : healthy I, healthy world! : the evolutionary practice of constructive consciousness or how to improve your life AND save our world / Gary Drisdelle.

Includes bibliographical references.
ISBN 978-0-9813861-0-2

   1. Conduct of life. 2. Health. 3. Happiness. I. Title.

BF637.C5D75 2010   158.1   C2010-901487-1

Printed in United States of America
First Edition

Disclaimer

The purpose of this book is to:

- inspire a calm and kind global practice of constructive consciousness for higher human potential

- recognize the weak control we have over our human nature and our inner mental programming

- clearly understand how to take control and stop our destructive habits

- support people in welcoming in a constructive and sustainable life of optimal health, enduring happiness, and peaceful prosperity

- encourage people to take care of themselves before helping others and the world

Even though the information presented in this book is believed to be true, useful, and as accurate as possible, it may have mistakes and does not cover all areas of constructive living. As with any information of this kind, individuals should do their own research on the ideas covered in this book and its extensions. All ideas, quotes, views, and other words written are intended without judgment toward any belief, individual or institution; if it seems otherwise it is completely unintended.

HealthyIsm, this book, the related websites, the author, and anyone else connected to this material in any way do not intend for any information, services, tools, or products to be used to diagnose, cure, treat, or prevent any disease or any medical condition or any other problem or non-problem. This book and the related websites shall be used by all at their own risk and discretion. This book does not endorse any method of recovery for habits, addictions, or compulsions of any kind.

This book, its contributors, and its extensions do not accept responsibility for any liability, harm, loss, damage, and/or any other reactions to, or for any use of, the information contained herein.

Captain of Your Ship

Before making any change in your life, especially in respect to the health of your body or mind, you should first check with an up-to-date, balanced, and licensed physician or primary health care provider.

Please note, only if you are of sound mind and you are *not* suffering from mental problems, that regardless of what *you* are diagnosed with and/or prescribed by a licensed health professional or anyone else, you are responsible for your own life. The onus is upon *you* to understand your body's needs and to welcome becoming your own personal expert on health, happiness, and prosperity, so that you can make important decisions about them. You must decide whether to follow any prescription, guidance, or advice you receive from other people or institutions. You are the captain in control of your vessel. You must assemble and manage your own crew of professionals—such as medical and complimentary doctors, teachers and mentors, fitness experts and nutritionists, and religious leaders and spiritual gurus—that will help you welcome your own optimal evolution that ultimately benefits all of us: Healthy *I,* Healthy World!

Dedication

To my family, who empower, endure, and endear me daily –
my children Kyle, Justyn, and Leigha
and especially my amazing life partner, Lekha

To my inspiring son who adopted me, Shayne

To my siblings and my dads, whom I love dearly –

To my extended family –
my sisters and brothers of the Earth community who are becoming aware of the factors that control them and are ready and willing to welcome optimally healthy, enduringly happy, and peacefully prosperous lives

And also, with much love, to yet another person becoming aware –
MYSELF

In Memory Of

In memory of my mother, Dolly;
In a primal way, I so sadly miss you, Mom.
But spiritually, I am so joyfully aware
That you simply exist in a different way

Love ya

Table of Contents

About This Book 1
Personal Declaration 11
Introduction 13

CONSIDERATION I: HealthyIst vs. Unhealthyolic 22
    Chapter 1.   What Is HealthyIsm? 23
    Chapter 2.   What Is an Unhealthyolic? 34
    Chapter 3.   Are You an Unhealthyolic? 40
    Chapter 4.   Is HealthyIsm Possible? 45

CONSIDERATION II: Seven Steps to HealthyIsm 59
    Chapter 5.   Step 1: What Happened to Us? 61
    Chapter 6.   Step 2: What's Your Current Truth? 100
    Chapter 7.   Step 3: Zoom Out – Review Your Overall Past....117
    Chapter 8.   Step 4: Zoom In – Reveal Your Messy Past 124
    Chapter 9.   Step 5: R.E.L.I.E.F.! 133
    Chapter 10.   Step 6: Develop Your HeLP 152
    Chapter 11.   Step 7: Support Your HeLP 199
    Chapter 12.   Quick Fix! 235

CONSIDERATION III: Receiving and Giving Support 245
    Chapter 13.   Welcoming In Support and Kindness 247
    Chapter 14.   Giving Out Support and Kindness 257

Appendix A.   Healthy I: I Am What I Do! 268
Appendix B.   Healthy World!: A Story of H.O.P.E. 280

Notes and Resources 305

About This Book

Welcome to the practice of HealthyIsm! If you are ready to stop destructive habits and develop constructive, healthy ones, then my greatest hope is that this book will inspire and support you as you do whatever it takes to calmly welcome a healthy, happy, and prosperous lifestyle. I am confident that, as more of us take control of our lives and regularly practice constructive consciousness, we will have a better chance to save the world from the mess of our past and present destructive ways. Yes, the focus of this book is a *healthy I,* but the ultimate goal is a *healthy world!* Because of the interconnectivity of all species and all other things on this vibrant biosphere called Earth, it is only through a sustainable healthy world that we can have the best chance of sustaining a healthy I.

The Genesis of HealthyIsm

To explain the genesis of this book and the practice of HealthyIsm, I must first share with you a bit of my personal history. Like most humans roaming this planet, I was programmed to be and think a certain way from the day I was born. As I grew, all the mental input from parents, friends, people, institutions, television, media, and so on formed the logic (and illogic) of my thinking process. Out of that thinking, along with instinctual urges, I made choices that shaped my reality, and some of those choices caused destruction in my life and, to some extent, contributed to the messed-up world we have today.

During my twenties I lived an easy life. I owned a rental property and did occasional handyman jobs which provided steady income. I also flew airplanes as a hobby, taught karate part time, drove nice cars and fast motorcycles, traveled the world over, had friends a-plenty and no shortage of girlfriends.

On the surface it looked like I had a great life, but underneath it all I often felt empty. Besides a reckless indulgence of junk food, drugs, alcohol, and frequent partying into the early hours of the morning, I also had a lonely secret life as a drug-smuggling mule. This *job* provided me with lots of extra cash, an abundance of drugs, and an addictive adrenaline rush every time I traveled with a hidden load of illicit substances. Eventually I got caught and was sentenced to several years in the American prison system. As a result, I lost everything, disappointed my friends, caused a lot of pain to my loved ones, and came very close to committing suicide.

As with most bad experiences, there are silver linings if one looks for them. The first short-term lining was that I survived my reckless choices; if I had not been caught I would have likely destroyed my health or been killed at some juncture in the ruthless drug-smuggling world. The long-term lining was that I went from losing everything to gradually rebuilding my life; discovering my special purpose on earth; studying fitness, nutrition, injury rehabilitation, life coaching, motivation, and general wellness; finding an amazing life partner; having beautiful children; and *legally* gathering resources to support all of this.

I became a healthy, happy, law-abiding guy who seldom got sick or emotionally down. Even with this new *clean* life, I continued to do various destructive things in my life, such as judging others, driving aggressively, ingesting too many daily treats like coffee and sweets, and too often indulging in marijuana and alcohol.

I had to take control. I needed to look within and outside myself to understand why I did what I did in the past and still did destructive things in the present.

I knew that if I recognized what caused my weaknesses and found ways to eliminate or control them, and improved my life in the process, I could share it with others and contribute to helping the world move beyond its destructive state of affairs. So, how could I improve my life and *save the world?* The best way that I could envision to do this was to develop an open-minded non-fanatical practice that was dedicated to constructive consciousness and improving one's life, then spreading the word by writing a book about it.

Since healthy can refer to body and mind and people's overall lifestyle, I chose to call this practice and the book *Healthy-Ism*. Just as vegetarianism is a focused practice of welcoming in a dedicated diet of predominantly plants, **HealthyIsm is simply a focused practice of calmly and kindly welcoming in the best possible levels of attainment in all areas of life.** The emphasized *I* in HealthyIsm symbolizes that a person must take care of oneself first before helping others or saving the world.

As I set out on this vision, I assumed it would be easy. "I'll finish writing in three months," I thought to myself. In the end, it took more than three years and turned out to be an enormous project. Not only did I have the tasks of researching, writing, publishing, and figuring out how to get the book out to the

3

world, I was also obliged to preach *only what I practiced*. But I was committed to bettering my life and helping the world. If you are reading this now, *and* it helps you in your life, then all of those tasks have indeed been accomplished.

Intent of This Book

The intent of this book is to encourage people to stop making a mess in their lives and the world. To do so, they can use the techniques offered within these pages or any method that pushes them to end their destructive thinking and actions and instead welcome a constructive life - be it help from religious or spiritual guidance, a loved one, a recovery group, a mentor, peer-to-peer support, a psychological or medical professional, a self-help method, a sudden awakening from some *aha* moment or a combination of any of these.

Please allow me to make it clear from the first: I am not a medical or psychological professional or a seasoned writer, and it is not my intention to tell people what to do with their lives. I am just a guy who loves and wants the evolutionary best for his earth, for his fellow humans and selfishly for his children. I am asking all people to consider taking a close look at what's going on inside and around them, recognize the weaknesses of human nature, and identify the thoughts—both their own and those of others—that may be largely responsible for leading them into an unhealthy, unhappy, deficient existence. This is not a book about positive thinking; it's about *constructive thinking and constructive functioning*.

This book and its correlating website, HealthyIsm.com, is intended to be a starting point for those who are ready and willing to take control of or improve their lives and, by extension directly or indirectly, help the world. Please note that just like an engineer presents her new design to the world even before it is "perfect", this book is also coming to you less than perfect. I welcome that, as you improve your life, you will also contribute to and improve the practice called HealthyIsm.

This book is intended only for reference and consideration and to provide support to people in their quest to welcome what humans are capable of, and what they yearn for, in their calmest and kindest state of mind—great health, happiness, and prosperity for self and for all. Through it, I hope to find a way to help the *I* in each of us, stop destructive lifestyle habits, and calmly and kindly embrace constructive habits such as:

- being aware of the weak control we have over human instincts and our inner mental programming
- relieving the negative controlling effects of this lack of control
- asking the "simple question" at all times: *Is this thought or action supportive (or at least neutral) to me, others, and/or the Earth, and does it ultimately welcome a calm and kind, healthy, happy, and prosperous evolution?*
- freeing the *I* from self-inflicted negative emotions
- offering permanent, unconditional forgiveness to self and others
- providing our bodies with just the right amount of proper nutrition
- keeping our bodies and minds free of harmful, destructive materials

- sufficiently using the muscles, nerves, bones, and other parts of our amazing bodies in the many physical ways for which they are intended
- being aware of our interconnection to others in one sense or another—that what you do for yourself, you do for others and vice versa
- participating once (or both times) in a brief, twice daily, simultaneous global meditation/prayer/focus of such reflections as unity, the present moment, a healthy I, and/or a healthy world
- finding ways to welcome in support and kindness
- finding ways to give out support and kindness

This is a proactive book that is mostly about what you *could* do, not what you *shouldn't* do. It is intended to spark something within you that makes you stand up, take charge of your life, and welcome in results. Above all, the HealthyIsm organization ventures out on this journey to set in place a support system of various resources that is all about giving the help that allows the greatest chance of success in that welcoming.

This book is about a practice called HealthyIsm—a call to recognize the weakness of our willpower to control the instinctual drives of our human nature and inner mental programming, to stop our destructive thoughts, habits, and actions, and to embrace a better life.

HealthyIsm is about helping oneself first, then helping or inspiring at least two other people as a way to both pass on the gift *and to reinforce what one is practicing*.

HealthyIsm is for those people who completely or partially lived destructive lifestyles in the past, not always by choice, but who are now ready and willing to embrace a constructive lifestyle. It is for those people who have experienced the pain of being unhealthy, unhappy, and deficient, who have suffered the consequences, who have learned a lesson or two, and who are ready to move on to a different approach.

The recurring principles in this book are based on the idea that any messes we find in ourselves and in our world are the result of two key potentially destructive forces: instincts and inner mental programming. These principles will be explored and expressed in different ways numerous times throughout the book as a method of driving the concepts into our brains—just like a coach repeats a certain drill or mantra until the athletes *get it*.

I acknowledge you and honor you for taking the time to focus on the I, for exploring this book, and perhaps for looking for a way to soften or eliminate your addiction to the unhealthy, unhappy, and deficient areas of your life—whatever those may be and in whatever degree they exist.

Using This Book

As you read this book please note that the parental upbringing, schooling, culture, political affiliation, social status, religious orientation, and beliefs and values of the reader are looked upon without judgment; if it seems otherwise it is completely unintended. This book merely asks you to step outside of yourself for a moment—and outside the control of any instincts or inner mental programming—to consider the implications or possibilities of those instincts and programming. Are they damaging in any way—either in the long or short term—to you, to others, or to our great Earth? If, logically or intuitively, you have even a hint that they are damaging, then the concept of HealthyIsm may be a practice to consider.

The information in this book is also offered *only for your consideration* and careful analysis. It is not meant to put down any person or institution or idea but rather to offer another way to look at reality and the way you think and act, and to offer ideas for trying something new that may lead you down the road toward an optimally healthy, peacefully productive, and enduringly happy life for yourself and for the rest of the world.

As novelist Dinah Mulock Craik famously said, "Believe only half of what you see and nothing that you hear." As you hear the words in this book, you are asked to research the information on your own and to use rational thinking and your intuition. You are asked to consider all information presented to you in the world as constructive or destructive to our evolution. Since you are merely asked to consider the information in this book, the sections are titled *Considerations*.

Consideration I looks at the contrast between a healthy, constructive lifestyle (HealthyIsm) and an unhealthy, destructive lifestyle, or life as an *Unhealthyolic*. You will also consider if you are an Unhealthyolic and ask yourself if you can welcome a life of health, happiness, and prosperity.

Consideration II lays out a seven-step method for stopping your Unhealthyolic habits by looking at how your "mess" began, identifying past messes that may dictate your present actions and habits, and finding ways to overcome these habits and welcome in a constructive lifestyle through the practice of HealthyIsm.

Consideration III provides a few more ideas for supporting and maintaining your new healthy, happy, and prosperous journey. It also looks at ways for you to be open to receiving and giving back to others, especially through showing by example.

This book and the HealthyIsm.com website will offer you ways to welcome becoming a "self-expert" in various areas, such as exercise, nutrition, spirituality, green living, adaptation to a changing world, and attaining and maintaining great health, happiness, and prosperity. Yes, it may take a little time to practice and understand how to become an expert—but practice is all it takes for us to learn anything new, like riding a bike or brushing our teeth or growing an organic garden or flying a space shuttle.

As you make your way through this book, may the aspects that are out of balance in your life, and that therefore do not support your optimal evolution, be immediately revealed to you in a kind and nurturing way, and never in a change-or-else way.

May you recognize any destructive aspects of your human nature, even if they served humanity well at one point in our evolution.

May all the programmers of your life be revealed so that you can understand how they have largely influenced the way you think and, thus, the way you live.

May this book gently assist you as you participate in surfing the wave of human awakening, seizing your thoughts, and embracing a life of HealthyIsm! If enough of us embrace this practice of constructive consciousness, we just may have a tiny side benefit of saving the world – wouldn't that be nice!

Personal Declaration

If you are ready and willing to stop your Unhealthyolic habits and welcome a life of optimal health, enduring happiness, and peaceful prosperity, sign this personal declaration as a commitment to your I to dedicate yourself to embracing a life of HealthyIsm. Simply acknowledge and check off the following promises to yourself to guide you as you read through this book.

I, _____ , do promise these things to myself:

☐ To be open to new ideas and habits

☐ To not be attached to any concepts suggested here

☐ To do my own research on concepts suggested here or elsewhere

☐ To apply the principles of HealthyIsm for at least 30 days

☐ To give my absolute best as I apply these principles

☐ To continually repeat the principles, 30 days at a time, if I see any signs of improvement in my health, happiness, and/or prosperity

☐ To face what I am and do, what habits I have, what I think and feel

- ☐ To love and accept myself as I am and to move forward at my own pace

- ☐ To always forgive myself as I am, and to forgive again if I slip up

- ☐ To ask for support if I am having a difficult time stopping unhealthy habits

- ☐ To support at least two other people who are ready and willing to change, once I am already committed to and welcoming a life of HealthyIsm

Commitment Pledge

(Write a personal statement of commitment, such as "I commit to all of the above" or "I commit to being free of my destructive habits and to instead welcoming a healthy, happy, and prosperous lifestyle—a life of HealthyIsm.")

I _____

_____

_____

_____

Signature: _____

Date: _____

Introduction

At the end of this book there is a futuristic story of alien scientists who visit earth around the year 2050 and despite observing chaos only a few decades earlier find the planet to be in a remarkably healthy state – the air is clean, the water pure, and the plants and animals vibrant. The scientists concluded that the humans, the dominant species who were also in excellent condition, had reached a critical point in their development where they had to choose between evolving or becoming extinct. Choosing life, they learned to cooperate with each other, created many good things as a network of communities, nurtured their planet, and as a result saved themselves.

Aliens aside, is this story of human self preservation and a healthy *new earth* possible or just wishful thinking? With so much daily *bad* news of sick people, a fragile environment, a volatile economy, widespread crime, oppressed and exploited sectors of society and of violent conflicts between regions, cultures, and religions and so on – how could we possibly have any form of control over this craziness and create such a future utopia? How? The answer lies within each one of us. The best hope for controlling the craziness *out there* in the world is to first manage what goes on *in here,* in our own lives. This book is dedicated to just that – finding ways to manage our lives, our thoughts and actions, so that we can exert our energies towards good, towards creating a balanced *utopia.* If enough of us start practicing higher consciousness in our personal worlds we can dramatically improve our collective world. The world is...*what I do*. Healthy I, healthy world!

All of these crises in the world have the power to be our potential destroyers; they also have the transformational power to be a giant evolutionary wakeup slap on the face of humanity that can snap all of us out of our spell of madness into a fresh state of calm awareness. With tears of virgin sanity each one of us must learn how to improve our own lives by practicing small *healthy* changes such as: eat a little better; consume a little less; smile a lot more; help a stranger; plant a small garden; pick up some trash; participate in a daily one minute global meditation, prayer, or focus (as described in the grey area on page 173); and so on. Then with momentum and boosted willpower go much bigger – forgive *everyone,* including ourselves, for *all* wrong doings (see Chapter 9); become experts on our bodies inside and out; help a nation; start a business that strives to do no harm; join others in using our strengths towards good, towards welcoming the things that we have to do, not only to survive but to flourish; and so on. If we look around and pay attention we can already find thousands of individuals and groups with great altruistic ideas that are showing us how we can flourish. *Now* is the time to use these crises/slaps as compelling reasons to control our minds, to choose life, to globally evolve into *constructively conscious humans.*

Homo Construttivo or whatever Latin name a new species of humans would be called, we collectively, either one at a time or as one, have to become aware of why we think and act the way we do, practice control, calmly and kindly keep doing the good things, courageously attend to the bad, and co-create the best that humans are capable of. Once we snap out of it, we have the capacity and the resources, such as shown in this book, to take care of most of the personal and global troubles we face today. Through centuries of collaborating ingenuity and good will, we have periodically harnessed constructive thinking to make our lives far safer and easier in various ways. Nowadays, like no other time in history, we often witness, participate in, or hear of positive news, of random acts of good will, of individuals and massive amounts of people from all walks of life, reaching out and taking care of each other *and* the planet. Human ingenuity has culminated in the development of computers and subsequently the Internet bringing with it many benefits to people's lives especially real-time communication and the decentralized, *unrestricted,* and global access to helpful knowledge.

As the numerous advantages of computers, the World Wide Web and other technologies continue to improve, multiply, and rapidly spread throughout the world, exponentially more of us are sharing wisdoms that are bringing a fresh insight into the multitude of human agendas that are negatively affecting our lives. Clusters of aware people everywhere are challenging their own destructive behaviors and instead welcoming human excellence. It's as if the constructive side of our collective consciousness has been forming, growing, and getting stronger while in a deep sleep, maturing to this era of a great awakening. As we open our eyes and look around, we are recognizing the aspects that have contributed to our crises. It's slowly but steadily becoming clearer how our inherited beliefs, views and values have held us back from our full potential and how a combination of nature and nurture had influenced—and continue to influence – our thoughts and actions. With the warmth and clarity of a slapped red face, it is time to practice constructive consciousness and take the actions necessary to evolve and welcome a strong and sustainable existence of great health, happiness, and prosperity (HHP).

Healthy *and* Happy *and* Prosperous

So what does it mean to be healthy *and* happy *and* prosperous within the practice of HealthyIsm?

- Healthy, the core of HealthyIsm, refers to an optimal state in *all* areas of one's life, especially having great physical and mental health to an old age. This means having at least the basic necessities of life (no, not chocolate or beer – although not to be denied), having a strong immune system to stave off illness, and having a stable mental chemistry to clearly make calm, kind, and constructive lifestyle choices.

- Happy means being in a state of *enduring* joy that has its foundation in *being one* with the present moment while having a grateful awareness of all the blessings in one's life. Lasting happiness is supported further by helping others whenever possible. There is a reason why we swell up with tears of compassionate joy when we hear a story of someone who was freely helped by a kind stranger to rise beyond his difficult circumstances in life. These tears are nature's way of saying that it's the right thing to do. Eating food when hungry brings a momentary smile; being *mindfully* grateful for the food produces a cheerful temperament, and helping to feed others in need brings enduring deep joy. Happiness is also enhanced by helping oneself to continuously grow and excel, not as a way to be better than others, but as an expression of human and evolutionary potential.

- Prosperous means having, in a kind, sustainable, and

peaceful way, the tools and resources to support health and happiness. Starting with gratitude for the greatest resource of all—one's thinking process—when welcoming in further tools and resources, all people, plants, and animals are treated fairly and compassionately with full awareness of the interconnection and interdependence of all things in the cycle *and* web of life.

In summary, when referring to HHP, it means optimally healthy, enduringly happy, and peacefully prosperous. But isn't it impossible for most people to have a life like this? Isn't our HHP dictated by our circumstances?

No! Our lives do not have to be dictated by our circumstances, no matter how difficult they may be. Instead, our HHP is largely dictated by the lack of awareness and weak control we have over our natural instincts and our inner mental programming (referred to as IMP), the resultant thoughts we think, and the actions we take! If we teach ourselves to be aware of our nature and our IMP and to train ourselves to welcome optimally healthy, enduringly happy, and peacefully prosperous life choices, then we can better influence a more constructive destiny for self and for all.

Evolving Humans

Human life is at the threshold of massive change, either through complete destruction or through an evolution to higher levels of consciousness. I believe, as do others, that we are headed to higher levels. Like an adolescent evolving to become less reckless and more responsible as he matures, society at large is maturing and evolving.

We are evolving spiritually by accepting globally, regardless of diverse backgrounds, that at the core of our very make-up is a common "mystery glue," an omnipresent, unprejudiced, unbiased, natural life force, source energy, God, consciousness or Universal Spirit that is in us and outside of us, that keeps our universe in place and that, at the same time, ties us all together in a sea of oneness.

We are evolving socially through enhanced communication, by being more aware of our connectivity to each other, by being more tolerant, kind, and compassionate, and by offering unconditional love and respect to ourselves and our diverse brothers and sisters of our mother earth. We are accepting that we must work together, as one, to clean up the many messes that we have made.

> ### Evolving Outside the Box of Conventional Science
>
> *The first law of thermodynamics says that energy cannot be created or destroyed. As has happened with many scientific laws throughout history, other scientists and researchers have tried to use, revise, prove otherwise, or completely quash this law with the goal of creating very cheap or even free energy. Regardless of whether these scientists revise the old laws or create new ones, free or very cheap power will revolutionize the world. There'd be no more fighting over oil; less of our labor and financial resources would go toward providing energy for our homes, cars, toys, greenhouses, and machines; and there'd be no pollution from the burning of fossil fuels. Our reliance on oil as the main source of energy has had a major influence on our IMP. The discovery and mass use of free, clean energy will be another positive step in the evolution of our planet.*

We are evolving scientifically by our individual and collective brain power, by welcoming ongoing constructive (not destructive) improvements for our life on earth that take all of us farther away from misery and pain and closer to a life of happiness and pleasure.

Science has either already created or is on the verge of creating amazing technologies like cheap or free energy, faster delivery of information on a global level, ethically and environmentally friendly consumer products, and bio- and nano-technology that will help to maintain or repair our bodies.

Slowly but surely, more and more of us are waking up to the reality of the destructive illusions and delusions that surround us every millisecond of every day. When enough people finally embrace a life of constructive consciousness,, they will have the power to help others transform their lives, too—first and foremost by showing by example.

If you are one of those early adopters of a life of Healthy-Ism and are feeling a bit lonely, don't worry! There is never a crowd on the leading edge, but the people will come once they see your healthy glow, your prosperous life, and your cheerful, stable attitude.

Taking the Reins

In her documentary *Humanity Ascending,* Barbara Marx Hubbard suggests that humans will either smother in a cocoon of destructiveness or catapult into the next stage, transcending as enlightened butterflies into something better than we could have ever imagined.[1] We are in the best position in the history

19

of humanity to transcend and take control of our IMP, our instincts, and our lives, but that opportunity can disappear soon enough, either through the destruction of our health or the health of our planet. As time goes by, it will become more difficult to take control, because our health is getting worse and worse—and with poor health comes foggy, desperate, and destructive thinking.

Today we live among extremes, with nations on one side exploding with obesity epidemics and nations on the other side starving to death. We face other epidemics of diabetes, poverty, suicide, obsession with thinness, obsession with possessions, and cancers of every part of the body.

Our mother earth is riddled with diseases in her forests and oceans caused by such other cancers as excessive human self-indulgence and lack of common sense. Our reckless use of resources—especially fossil fuels—is destroying our earth and our health. It's as if we are all sitting in a massive global garage with our cars and smokestacks billowing out poisons, unwilling to turn them off, blithely saying with labored breath that everything is okay or it's not our problem.

Isn't it obvious that something is not working? We have to wake up and recognize all our destructive instincts and our IMP!

If a person is standing on the edge of a building ready to commit suicide, isn't there always a huge effort to save that person? Isn't that person always calmly and kindly encouraged to reflect and delicately told that nothing is worth taking one's own life? Perhaps it's time for us to do the same with our own lives and our own planet: that as we stand on the edge of destroying our health and the health of the earth, we collectively decide that all the "destructive" sides of our thinking and actions are simply not worth it.

When we finally make the shift from Unhealthyolic to HealthyIsm, it will be as a result of the awareness of our instincts and our IMP, of all our thoughts and actions—such as an awareness that we only need so much and that, as consumers, every purchase we make has an effect on our own evolution and the evolution of all. For the longest time, people simply didn't know any better. But now we do. We are living in the time of an awareness revolution. We not only know what to do to live a constructive life but also how to go about it and how to overcome our destructive habits. There is no excuse anymore! It's time for gathering information, careful consideration, and constructive action.

CONSIDERATION I

HealthyIst vs. Unhealthyolic

In this first Consideration, we will introduce you to HealthyIsm and set the foundation for the next Considerations by addressing several questions:

- What is HealthyIsm?
- What is an Unhealthyolic?
- How did we get to such an unhealthy and destructive place?
- Are you an Unhealthyolic?
- Is HealthyIsm possible?
- How can we achieve a healthy and constructive condition?

This section is also about introducing you to how our inner mental programming (IMP) has taken over our lives and rules our health, happiness, and peaceful prosperity. We will touch on how our instincts, which at one time we relied upon for survival and evolution—are now partly to blame for the destructive condition of the individual, the human collective, and our great mother earth.

Please take note: reading and applying what follows in this book will enable you to change your life (for the better, of course)—so if you are ready and willing, let's begin.

What Is HealthyIsm?

Transcend personal pride, honor human achievement.
—Idea from David Hawkins
Power vs. Force

HealthyIsm is not about defending against the negative stuff of self and the world. It IS simply the practice of stopping destructive habits and welcoming in what most people yearn for in their calmest and kindest thoughts…
—Gary Drisdelle, *HealthyIsm*

The first wealth is health.
—Ralph Waldo Emerson

HealthyIsm, in its shortest definition, is simply the practice of stopping destructive Unhealthyolic habits and welcoming in optimal health, enduring happiness, and peaceful prosperity (HHP).

HealthyIsm in its entirety is the loving practice of calmly and kindly, *and at one's own pace,* respecting one's own *self* by becoming aware of the weak control we have over our destructive instincts and inner mental programming, then finding ways to stop that destructiveness and welcome what most people yearn for in their calmest and kindest state of mind, which is great HHP for self, for others, and for the world

Healthy I, Healthy World!

The emphasized *I* in HealthyIsm underscores the idea that those who practice it focus, *by choice,* first on taking care of themselves—just as in an aircraft emergency a person would first put on his own oxygen mask before helping others. Their ultimate goal is to help the world, through bettering the *I,* to calmly and kindly evolve into an optimally healthy, enduringly happy, and peacefully prosperous place: healthy *I,* healthy world!

Practicing HealthyIsm means looking at the health of the planet and understanding that we, humans of the global tribe, who are all part of a living organism called Earth, have an important biological and psychological role and that we are an inseparable part of its celestial body: what we do for or against our planet, we ultimately do for or against ourselves. What we do for ourselves, good or bad, we do for our planet and all its inhabitants. The practice of HealthyIsm suggests that for a healthy world we must start by *doing good for ourselves.*

HealthyIsm can be found everywhere; it crosses all lines of geography, religion, ethnicity, social status, and politics. Just as vegetarianism can thrive in China or Canada, among the Jewish or Catholic, among the gay or straight, so too HealthyIsm can thrive in Brazil or France, among Muslims or Buddhists, among male or female. HealthyIsm has no boundaries.

Practicing HealthyIsm is *not* limited to the methods described in this book; people are encouraged to use any calm and kind approach that stops destructive habits and replaces them with constructive ones.

HealthyIsts

People who practice HealthyIsm—HealthyIsts, in fact—are people who have the habit of being optimally healthy, enduringly happy, and peacefully prosperous, and who welcome a constructive lifestyle without concern for the judgment, acceptance, or denial of others.

HealthyIsts do not waste energy worrying about what others think. They know that, without being fanatical, all their thoughts and actions are intended for the betterment of themselves, of all mankind, and of our planet. They aim to live in harmony with and as close to nature as possible.

HealthyIsts realize that many manmade creations such as television, big league sports, the Gregorian calendar, credit based monetary system, and various technologies serve our needs but more often than not, because of habit or ignorance, we become their slaves. When various creations weaken our personal power we call them illusions and will either avoid them our use them rationally, wisely, and responsibly. If HealthyIsts find that an illusion is using them, they will take corrective action.

For example, a HealthyIst may use a computer to research a topic of interest, pay some bills, write a book, communicate with others, or even play a game or two for entertainment. But he will strive to limit his time in front of the computer to a *healthy* amount. If the "gigabytes are biting" and he finds himself obsessed with the beautiful array of functions that a computer offers, he will take action to regain control, perhaps using methods like those offered in this book.[2] Perhaps he will make time to

> ### Let the Children Grow
>
> *If only all the children of the world were allowed to grow from birth with full love and ample nutrients, and were kept from toxic chemicals and the destructive IMP, we would likely have a constructive, global tribe and a peaceful, healthy world. If only we nurtured them with the attributes of awareness, acceptance, forgiveness, oneness, being proactive, and giving and receiving pure calm and kind support, the children could develop in a constructive, natural way from the moment of birth. If only, unless absolutely necessary, they were never drugged (except for the drug of love) or fed processed food. If only, as they grew, they were allowed to explore, hunt, play, and be curious and giddy without a thousand unnecessary no's or any fear of impatience from their aware parents. If only they were recognized as an expanding, evolutionary, biological process—just as a flower naturally blooms and withers—with the pure intention of an unimpeded cycle of life.*
> *It's time to let the child in all of us grow to the highest potential!*

get away from the screen and do something related to nature, like taking a walk in the woods or park, by himself or with others, taking in the sunshine, pondering and meditating on the immense beauty all around him. He may spend his meditative time aware of his own breath and pulse and envisioning his connection to all other things natural, including the earth below and the stars and planets of the universe above.

That same HealthyIst recognizes that indulging in any product can present an occasional stumbling block. He may have a glass of wine with supper, for example, using the wine to enhance the flavor of the meal and support pleasant feelings. But if he constantly craves that feeling and finds himself polishing off a full bottle night after night, he knows that there is an imbalance and that the illusion is using him. He once again takes the hint to regain control.

HealthyIsts acknowledge their way of thinking, their inner mental programming, in all manners in which it has been presented or offered to them (any creed, constitution, religion, special ability, and so on) and welcome their absolute best with this divine gift of thought; this is their starting point. They accept their biology in every way, from their physical makeup to the primal movements of walking, running, pulling, pushing, climbing, twisting, and throwing. They do not judge, victimize, discriminate against, or shame themselves or others. They replace this way of thinking by welcoming tolerance, patience, love, and kindness.

They are people who have embraced their world, culture, and schooling for all the gifts that they offer, like love, courage, knowledge, identity, imaginative arts, music, and dance, perseverance, and community. They smile and forgive the immature and irrational destructive forces of others' beliefs, as well as their own, which have caused and continue to cause much of the strife and destructiveness that exist in our society today.

They realize that there is much craziness in the world, both in the past and now, in the present. They are aware that there are many world issues to deal with immediately and simultaneously, and they know that the best way to start solving those issues is to first help themselves to recognize and recover from their own Unhealthyolic habits. They know they must first create a healthy *I* and then, as if through a ripple effect, help and inspire others to do the same. Healthy I, healthy world.

> **What HealthyIsm Is Not!**
>
> *HealthyIsm is not selfish or effortless. It is not an expectation of others. It is not about pointing fingers. It is not propaganda, nor eugenics, nor state intervention, nor a money-sucking, get-healthy-and-happy-quick scheme. HealthyIsm is not limited to the methods in this book! It is not a forced belief system, nor is it a cult or a religion. It is not closed to helpful ideas, nor closed in by borders or boundaries, nor elitist, nor a judgment of big business, governments, religion, culture, or media. It is not meant to be "in your face."*
>
> *HealthyIsm is not about defending against the negative stuff of self and the world. It IS simply the practice of stopping destructive habits and welcoming in what most people yearn for in their calmest and kindest thoughts—HHP for self and all.*

Acts of Kindness

HealthyIsts are aware of the challenges in the world; at the same time, they are aware of the positive signs around them. As the Dalai Lama once said, there are more acts of kindness going on in the world today than ever before in the history of humankind. For example, WiserEarth.com, a website dedicated to listing and connecting social justice and environmentally friendly people and groups, estimates that there are more than *one hundred thousand* organizations around the world *and* millions of individuals working toward a better, healthier earth.

> *Equal Voices*
>
> *What will it take to allow all people, especially women, to freely evolve and be involved in all aspects of our global home? A sustainable, healthy, happy, prosperous, and peaceful world will become a reality sooner if both genders are allowed to have an equal voice and power on the local and world stages. Many countries have accepted women as part of their governing and corporate bodies, but even those have a long way to go. Women worldwide are awakening to the oppression they've endured for millennia, and they're ready for change. They are just now becoming involved in areas like decision-making and controlling their own fertility, and are an important part of our collective recovery from a destructive, unbalanced, "man"-made path. Equality will happen through the awareness and control of the destructive forces of human nature and the IMP that resides in both males and females that dictates our unfair thoughts and actions. Let's take control and allow the beauty of all to evolve and be equal.*

Here is another example in which, if all the information on the Internet represents the predominant thinking of a modern world, the numbers are quite interesting: in August 2004 I performed searches on a series of positive words, along with their opposite negative words, to see what was happening on the web. The word *hate* showed up on 6.8 million web pages. I thought that was a disheartening number until I found that the word *love* was on 42 million pages. *Evil* showed up on 7.7 million pages, *good* on 66 million, and so on. Today, five years later, the ratio is the same. Does this small sampling of search terms represent a world filled with more thoughts of kindness and goodness than of their negatives?

In the chaos of the times we live in, there is always an emergence of a so-called positive and a negative. Perhaps we have already reached our negative capacity and we can now begin the times of the positive. Perhaps society is maturing and becoming more rational, wiser, and more ready for calm, joy, and peace.

Despite their optimism, HealthyIsts are tempted by their IMP and instincts to react to the many world challenges with anger and sadness—but in the end they hold back, breathe into the moment, become present, accept what is, forgive all, and simply ask themselves: *What thoughts and actions are needed to first improve myself and only then to help improve, calmly and kindly, this situation?*

Web and Cycle of Life

HealthyIsts embrace the web and cycle of life. They are able to grasp their interconnectivity and interdependence with all things and also the fact that there is no waste in nature. If so inclined, some consider that when their physical bodies die, their souls or essence may evolve and come back again or remain *at home* with their Universal Spirit/God. They know that their bodies, if buried directly in the ground with no coffin, would decompose and be used by the earth in myriad ways to feed the web of living things and to create the cycle once again.

If nature chooses to end a HealthyIst's life, she accepts her fate with love and ease. HealthyIsts may feel rational sadness about leaving loved ones behind, but they do not fear death. If a HealthyIst loses a loved one, she may feel a primal yearning for that person and mourn from the deepest part of her core, but mentally she will not succumb to the anguish and depression exacerbated by her IMP. Instead she will become stronger, using the death as a catalyst for better things, and will keep welcoming or maintaining her HHP.

HealthyIsts embrace their bodies with or without clothing, though they may have been civilly trained to cover their bodies. They find no shame in walking naked at home among family or on a nude beach, taking in the healthy rays of the sun. But they do not force their bodies in their natural state on others, and they cover up when appropriate. They are also aware of the dangers of the environment and take precautions to protect their bodies against wind, cold, heat, unhealthy vegetation, contaminated air, and overexposure to the sun. They put the health of their own bodies and, by extension, the health of the earth first.

HealthyIsts spend their lives in abundance and build their prosperity by creating tools, products and services that are sustainable and constructive to the earth and her inhabitants, or that are at least neutral. They know how to serve others without selfishness. They understand that they are just a drop in the giant, infinite, and eternal holographic ocean of oneness and that they are, indeed, also serving themselves.

Yes, we HealthyIsts are optimists—not blindly, but backed by a lot of evidence of a humanity maturing and waking up to the reality of all things around us. We are tapping into a new power stronger than any nuclear reactor or star—the power of constructive aware living, such as practiced within HealthyIsm.

All actions and thoughts of HealthyIsts, which reach into the compassionate element of the human brain, are at least neutral to self or others and most often add to the recipe of human goodness. As David Hawkins shows in his inspiring book Power vs. Force, historically, humanity has been roaming around in the lower levels of consciousness where shame, grief, fear, and aggression reside. It is only in the twentieth century that humanity has begun to move to the higher levels of courage, acceptance, reason, love, joy, peace, and, eventually, beyond.[3] If you are reading this book, then you are probably at least in the higher level of courage: the courage to make changes, stop destructive habits, and welcome goodness into your life.

As a human being, you are by nature a creative survivor. When you are in your top form, benefiting from awareness and wisdom, you live your life enjoying the moment and welcoming in your deepest constructive impulses, which are toward growth, unity, and love. When you choose to live at these supportive levels, you are living a life of HealthyIsm.

Proof of Our Oneness?

In the world of quantum physics, what Einstein called "spooky action at a distance" perhaps rests the case of oneness. Researchers have shown that one electron can be in two places at the same time. Amazingly, what happens to an electron in one location happens at the exact same time to that electron in another location. Does this indicate we are all part of one body?[4]

By taking blood samples from all known ethnic groups around the world, geneticist Spencer Wells shows in his "single origin" hypothesis that all humans originated from the same tribe in Namibia. Are we all part of one family?[5]

For many, the concept of oneness is hard to believe. But if everyone absolutely knew it to be true, saw proof, AND believed it—that we are all part of the same thing, all connected as one big body and one big family—it's very likely that, almost overnight, we would collectively stop our destruction and calmly welcome in HHP.

But forget about "proof" just for a moment and instead just "imagine" our connectivity. Just as people act out their lives because they accept as true various dogmas and beliefs, imagine for a moment that we all believed, even without absolute proof, that we are all one…just imagine.

What Is an Unhealthyolic?

2

Thinking is the most unhealthy thing in the world, and people die of it just as they die of any other disease.
—Oscar Wilde

*As I wake up and come to know what is real and what is an illusion, I find my little destructive behaviors falling by the wayside, such as taking out my occasional frustrations on my husband. Instead I take out the garbage...
the garbage in my head, that is.*
—Lekha Lutchmansingh

In a disordered mind, as in a disordered body, soundness of health is impossible.
—Cicero

Now that we have an idea of what HealthyIsm is and what a HealthyIst is, let's take a look at the other side—the Unhealthyolics. Simply put, Unhealthyolics are individuals who cannot stop or change their destructive behaviors, regardless if they are aware or unconscious that those behaviors may be immediately or eventually damaging to themselves or others.

Unhealthyolics are people who have harmful dependencies, habitual tendencies, compulsions, and addictions to various destructive lifestyle practices that they won't—or feel they *can't*—give up. Sometimes it's a matter of not wanting to "sacrifice" their cigarettes, predatory business dealings, wine, joints, or prescription drugs. Other times it's seemingly harmless thoughts and actions that identify an Unhealthyolic, such as judgment of others, perpetual laziness, excessive use of earth's resources or consumption of destructive foods.

If they *are* aware of their destructive behaviors and admit to being Unhealthyolics, then they are one step closer to taking control and having more constructive lives *if they so choose.*

The choice to do as we please with our own bodies is debated as a basic human right, but let's face it: we are not doing our lives or the welfare of the world justice by interfering with our most basic natural needs. The minds and bodies that nature bestowed on us work best when provided with sufficient and proper nutrients, exercise, play, social interaction, sunshine, and so on, and are not meant to be tampered with in the way that we've been doing in our lifetime and even for hundreds, and thousands, of years.

Humans, like the rest of the animal kingdom, require specific ingredients for an optimal existence. A not-so-funny fact is that no other animals eat unhealthy foods or gain weight from lack of exercise (except for our domesticated pets), have destructive belief systems, become overly docile, disrespect the land they live on, exploit others, use drugs or alcohol, over-consume, or harm themselves, others, or the earth unnecessarily.

Unhealthyolics are people who continue to think destructive thoughts and give into destructive instincts even after they witness the harmful results of such thoughts and instincts. Some may ask, *But what about the man who was never sick or unhappy, who drank a bottle of whiskey and smoked a pack a day, who lived until the age of 92? Isn't our longevity determined by our genes?*

Well, first of all, had that man lived a more constructive life, he might have lived healthily and happily until the age of 122! Sure, on the surface it looked like he had fun in his life, indulging in his desires and living *for* the moment, but did he drink and smoke because he was having fun or because it reminded him of the fun he had in his youth or was he escaping horrible memories and aspects of his present reality? Secondly, though his actions seemed to not have affected *him* adversely, they likely caused great harm or illness to others around him and contributed to a messy world.

When we live *for* the moment we often hunger for a physical, mental or emotional fix of some sort, often trading negative consequences for fleeting pleasures. An occasional recreational fix may be inconsequential, and may bring brief smiles and warm memories of that moment. But when we move beyond recreational into habitual cravings we become negligent to our bodies, exploit life, and excessively consume things that we do not need physically or mentally. In doing so we either deplete our bodies of the essentials needed to be healthy or we overwhelm our physical and mental systems unnecessarily with excessive stressors/garbage.

If we lean toward optimal, healthy, happy, and constructive conscious choices, while living *in* the moment, accommodating all of our biological needs, our undesirable genetic predispositions will have a better chance of remaining unlocked and unable to come out. Our genetic predisposition does not have to be our destiny! On the contrary, our genetic destiny will largely be dictated by the ongoing conscious control we have over the destructive instincts of our human nature, the thoughts we think, and the actions we take.

People Aren't the Only Unhealthyolics

Unhealthyolics also come in the form of the world's governments, religious organizations, corporations, educational systems, and customs that also act from a destructive instinct and IMP place. These institutions and traditions, perhaps blindly, are often allowed to "do the thinking" for the majority of the population, and ultimately promote their Unhealthyolic addictions to the people, who then take harmful actions as a result. How do they continue to do it? Are we so powerless against them?

It's actually quite simple. It takes time for a child to develop to an age when he or she can use reasoning and rational thinking to eliminate Unhealthyolic habits and make constructive choices, such as using proper social manners or choosing to eat mostly healthy foods instead of too much sugary stuff. The same can be said for the world and its people as a whole. We, the global tribe, with free access to knowledge, are just now beginning to mature to a point where we recognize how lack of control over our instincts and thinking has been and still is causing the sickness, recklessness, and destruction in us and around us. Through immature and unaware thinking, individuals, institutions, and traditions as a whole up until now have created many illusions that caused a deficiency or toxicity to our health and the health of our planet. Then they passed that deficiency on to their followers, subordinates, citizens, employees, or students. It's time for all people and institutions to take a close look—a very close look—at what's going on around them, and to identify the internal and external Unhealthyolics who are living an existence of destructive lifestyle choices. Such scrutiny is essential for the individual and the world in order to evolve beyond the craziness of our *modern* day.

Beyond Control?

In our wonderful but habitually wicked world a destructive life seems sometimes beyond an individual's control. A person may live in a toxic household, be unable to control her environment, be forced to endure destructive acts day after day, or have no house at all. She may be oppressed by a dictatorial regime or even brainwashed and controlled by a so-called democratic government that is influenced by the agendas of a privileged few. She may have grown up with parents and a culture that knew no better. She may also have to work in unhealthy conditions just to feed herself and her family. Or, because she has kids, she may feel stuck with a self-absorbed, high-powered executive spouse or a self-abusing spouse who sits around lazily all day watching TV, spending rent money on pizza, beer, pot and cigarettes.

Of course there are some people with complex mental illnesses and life circumstances who need the help of medical professionals or others who can offer much more than the scope of this book. With those exceptions, most ready and willing individuals can improve their lives dramatically by being aware of their mental manipulators, then practicing control, changing the way they think, and calmly and kindly welcoming an HHP lifestyle. Easier said than "thunk," yes, but it can and *has* been done by many, many people from all walks of life and of *all* different circumstances and abilities.

In summary, an Unhealthyolic is an individual (or institution) who has the capability of being constructive in life but who still succumbs to destructive instincts and IMP and consequently does damaging things to himself, others, and the great earth.

Maybe you've been asking yourself, *Am I an Unhealthyolic?* The next chapter will delve into that question and ask you to do a little soul-searching to find out where you fall in the healthy/unhealthy spectrum.

> *"Man is made or unmade by himself; in the armory of thought he forges the weapons by which he destroys himself; he also fashions the tools with which he builds for himself heavenly mansions of joy and strength and peace."*
>
> —James Allen, *As a Man Thinketh*

3 Are You an Unhealthyolic?

If addiction is judged by how long a dumb animal will sit pressing a lever to get a "fix" of something, to its own detriment, then I would conclude that "net news" is far more addictive than cocaine.
—Rob Stampfli

If you do anything long enough to escape the habit of living, the escape becomes the habit.
—David Ryan

Sickness is the vengeance of nature for the violation of her laws.
—Charles Simmons

Don't worry—the *-olic* part of Unhealthyolic is not meant to have the same connotation of "disease" that a word like alcoholic does. It is simply meant as a nudge to wake ourselves up, recognize that there is a problem, and ask ourselves if we can do better when it comes to HHP.

An Unhealthyolic is a person who thinks thoughts or takes actions that are destructive to themselves, to others or to the Earth. If you're asking yourself if you're an Unhealthyolic, then there is a possibility that you are—especially if you read the Table of Contents and came straight to this page!

But if you're still not sure, ask yourself these questions:

- Am I unaware of my destructive instincts and my IMP that shape the way I think and act?
- Am I unaware of how others continue to influence my unhealthy and destructive habits?
- Have I ever felt the need to change my destructive behaviors?
- Has my doctor or health professional ever told me to change my destructive ways—and I haven't?
- Do I ever feel guilty about thoughts or actions that are destructive to self or others, directly or indirectly, like regularly consuming unhealthy foodstuff or yelling at a loved one?
- Do I exploit others or misuse the earth's resources even if there are many viable alternatives?
- Do I regularly need numerous coffees or other stimulants every day just to function or feel good?
- Am I an angry and/or dangerous driver willing to jeopardize my life and the lives of others by speeding, cutting

people off, and running red lights?
- Do people who talk to me about wellness, being constructive, creating abundance, sustainability, or HealthyIsm annoy me?
- Do I have a general negative gut feeling about many things I do in life?
- Am I emotionally upset and do I feel continuous anger, sadness, or guilt about the past or present?
- Do I worry about the future?
- Am I showing signs of preventable diseases that could be healed through good lifestyle choices?
- Do I keep gaining at someone else's loss?
- Do I have a constant craving for drugs (legal and illegal) or alcohol?
- Do I have a constant desire to shop and buy things that I don't really need?
- Are my stress levels off the chart?
- Am I unaware of or lost in the manmade construct of time?
- Do I instinctively know that things need to change in my life, but I don't have the willpower or energy to change them?
- Do I still eat certain foods even if I know they leave me feeling weak, sick, and/or bloated?
- Has my spouse lovingly "encouraged" me to change, but I feel sad, helpless, or annoyed by it?
- Do I use a company's products or services even when I have an intuition or a complete awareness that the company's products and dealings are not good for humans or the earth?
- Do I still smoke even though my lungs hurt or I have a persistent cough?
- Do I often find myself getting annoyed with my children?

- Do I interpret reality as others have taught me or as I see it on television shows, major news stations, reality shows, and other media?
- Do I have an overwhelming desire to acquire material goods just to keep up with—or outdo—the Joneses next door?
- Do I already live a good lifestyle but still feel the need to work more hours and make more money—all at the expense of a balanced lifestyle in which I could spend more time with my family or with myself?
- Does making eye contact with another human being make me feel uncomfortable?
- Do I deny my connection to others as co-inhabitants of the physical earth and/or as spiritual beings?
- The simple question: *Do my thoughts, actions, or goals ultimately take me, others, and/or the earth farther away from a calm and kind, constructive, healthy, happy, and prosperous evolution?*
- Am I an Unhealthyolic?

All the above scenarios have something in common: they are all thoughts and actions that do not kindly, calmly, and constructively support your evolution or the evolution of others or of the earth. If you answered yes to any of these questions, you can say that you are an Unhealthyolic.

If you determined that you are *not* an Unhealthyolic—good for you! But be careful—make sure you asked those questions to your rational, mature mind and not your destructive instincts or IMP, which may be masking the truth. If you determined that you *are* an Unhealthyolic, however—well, that's good news, too. Being conscious of a weakness is half the battle of correcting that weakness. So congratulations for coming this far! Remember that you are not being told that you *must* let go of your unhealthy habits; maybe you like them and you're happy the way you are. But I bet that if you are reading this book, then you are indeed looking for change.

The next chapter questions whether HealthyIsm is possible and looks at areas such as – why take control of our lives, having an open mind and especially defining your personal compelling reason to change

Is HealthyIsm Possible?

*Whether you believe you can or believe you can't,
you are right.*
—Henry Ford

*Go confidently in the direction of your dreams.
Live the life you have imagined. As you simplify your life,
the laws of the universe will be simpler.*
—Henry David Thoreau

*That which we are, we are…
and if we are ever to be any better,
now is the time to begin.*
—Alfred Lord Tennyson

Is HealthyIsm possible? Can you control your human nature and mind and become optimally healthy, enduringly happy, and peacefully prosperous? Can you become constructive in your life? Yes, you can! With enough knowledge, resources, and good reasons, absolutely anyone can become a HealthyIst and begin living a life of HealthyIsm. The first step is to simply become aware of destructive instinctual drives and inner mental programming (IMP) and seize control of your own mind!

Taking Control

We have tons of toys and conveniences in our lives, yet we are less happy and have less time to make ourselves happy. Depression is everywhere. Destruction is everywhere. Why is that? It's because we are unaware of destructive instinctual drives and the control that the IMP has over us. This disconnects us from our beautiful authentic nature-selves and the experience of living in the present moment. Many of us are stuck in the programming of our past and stress and worry about the future. We need to monitor our instincts and IMP to take control of our mental manipulators and learn to be the directors, not the directed.

Our DNA is not the sole determinant of our health. Nor do social, religious, racial, or other factors determine how healthy, happy, and prosperous we will or will not be. Yes, those influences can make it harder on us in some cases, but so many people from all sorts of different "starting places" go on not only to live in optimum health, happiness, and prosperity (HHP), but also to inspire and encourage others from all walks of life to improve their own situations.

Why do some people continue their destructive lifestyles and

> **Can We Control Our Minds?**
>
> *You betcha! In fact, we do it all the time, though not always for healthy reasons.*
>
> *Consider the case of Aron Ralston, a young man hiking alone in the Grand Canyon. At some point, a boulder fell and pinned his forearm. Unable to move for five days, he finally made the life-saving decision to cut off his own hand…with a dull pocket knife! Just think of the control he had to have over his mind, first to come to that wrenching decision, and then to overcome the physical and emotional pain he was surely experiencing.*
>
> *That may be an extreme example, but it just goes to show the power we humans can exert over our own minds when we want or need to. If you are ready and willing, you have the power to cut your Unhealthyolic habits and welcome a life of sustainable HHP!*

others don't? One could say it's the result of the inner mental programming of their culture or of the influence of parents, peer pressure, follow-the-herd mentality, media brainwashing, or even genetics—but at the root of it all, it's about unawareness. We don't know *that we don't know*. We are *unaware* that we *don't* know about our destructive instincts and IMP and how they manipulate our minds. But that's okay; let's forgive ourselves and welcome in awareness, which we can do by practicing HealthyIsm.

Becoming a HealthyIst doesn't mean that you'll have perfect health, enjoy great prosperity, or be eternally happy. However, it does mean that you'll be better positioned to be more constructive in your life.

You'll find that as you practice HealthyIsm and take more and more beneficial actions, it'll become easier and easier to be healthy, happy, and prosperous.

As an added comfort, consider this: as you enjoy the benefits of becoming constructive in your life you will also be leading the way not only for those in your immediate family and but also for people far and wide including those you have never met! Others will feel more empowered to embrace HealthyIsm just because someone else, someone like you, has already started practicing. It's as if every person who clears a path through the jungle of unawareness and destructive illusions—and welcomes improved HHP—clears the way for many others to follow.

Why wait until your body starts hurting or the doctor tells you that you have problems? Take control now and design a constructive life! Even the smallest improvements in making constructive mental choices have huge benefits. No matter how bad your life is right now, you still have the ability to improve at least a little—and by doing so, there is the likely chance that you will set in motion the ability to improve dramatically.

Why Take Control?

We must take control so we can constructively participate in a common, healthy future. The goal of HealthyIsm is to become aware of the mental manipulators in your life and to no longer let your thoughts, or the thoughts and actions of others either past or present, dictate your health, happiness, and prosperity. Once you start steering your own ship, here is what will happen:

- You'll be able to look at all the instinctual impulses and

programmed influences that come your way and decide for yourself whether to welcome them or control them.
- You'll begin to look at food as your best medicine for physical and mental health, and an ingredient for happiness and prosperity.
- You'll begin to properly use your body for what it was designed for—movement!
- You'll live in the now and be mindful of your every thought and breath—another essential ingredient of HHP.
- You'll have stronger constructive, loving, and forgiving relationships with self and others.
- You'll begin to develop and maintain the resources, tools, and assets that will help you welcome in greater HHP.
- You'll experience a constant high-energy "buzz"—or "high" or "euphoria", or whatever you want to call it—because your body and mind will be strong and clear.
- You'll feel amazing every morning, with loads of energy, a clear mind, and no need for coffee or sweets to wake you up. You might indulge on occasion to create warm feelings and memories, but only if you are already healthy and in control.
- You'll look amazing, too. It may take a few months to cleanse your body of the effects of destructive habits, but eventually people will wonder what miracle pill you're taking!

And you can tell them it's the pill of HealthyIsm.

Personal Compelling Reason to Change

Before embarking on the seven steps to stopping destructive

habits, it's essential that you first take a few moments to consider *why* you want to change. Having a *compelling and personal reason* for wanting to break bad habits will give you more focus, more energy, more motivation, and more desire as you start your journey to HealthyIsm. What's your motivation?

Get out a clean sheet of paper and jot down what it is that is pushing you to make a change. If you need some help, take a look at the following list of statements and circle anything that stands out for you.

I want to make a change because

- I want a better world.
- It's a matter of life or death.
- I've had a small taste of healthy behavior, I liked it, and I want more of it.
- I just had a baby or found out I/we are pregnant.
- I want to set an example for my children.
- I want to set an example for the world.
- I feel burned out, depressed, or apathetic.
- there's a conflict between my desire for HHP and my destructive habits.
- I had an epiphany—a sudden understanding, moment of clarity, or realization that I have to change.
- my health is deteriorating.
- I'm unhappy.
- I saw someone else looking healthy and happy.
- I saw someone else who used to be unhealthy and has now improved or changed.
- I'm having a mid-life crisis.
- I have too much stress.

- I'm bored.
- I want more of something.
- it can't get any worse.
- I've reached rock bottom; there's no place to go but up.
- I have new knowledge and awareness.
- I'm ready to move to the next level.
- I just realized that I am in control.
- I want to maximize my potential.
- I want recognition.
- I did some soul searching.
- I came to a shocking realization.
- I feel ashamed.
- I fear the alternative.
- I hate my life.
- I love the alternative.
- I love my life.
- I sense that there is a global shift, a need to do better as an individual and as a whole.
- I have a heightened awareness, due to some experience, of the need to take care of me.
- I accept that it's time.
- I simply decided, for no apparent reason, that I want to change.
- I want to attain (or help others attain) the basic hierarchy of needs and beyond: physiological needs, safety, love, belonging, confidence, achievement, self-actualization, and transcendence.

Did you choose one of the above statements or come up with something else as your compelling reason to change? Did you notice that all the reasons above are *personal?* That's because your reason *must be* personal. If you make a change for someone else, it simply won't work—or if it does, it probably won't stick for long. A mother pulling her overweight teenager to an exercise class will likely not succeed in getting the child to change. Change must come from

> *Strong reasons make strong actions.*
> —William Shakespeare

within, so your reason for making that change must be strong enough, compelling enough, and personal enough to motivate you and keep you on the path.

Take another look at this compelling personal reason you came up with. On a scale of 1 to 10 (with 1 being "no desire to change" and 10 being "strong desire to change *now*"), what would you say is your intensity level when you think about your reason? *If your intensity level is 6 or below,* you might want to tweak your reason to make it stronger or find a more compelling reason to overcome destructive habits.

Remember that the higher the intensity level, the higher your motivation to change—and the better the chance that you'll stick to a more constructive way of living.

An Open Mind

In becoming HealthyIsts we are asked to consider alternative ways of thinking that call into question the accepted beliefs and science upon which our current societal model is based.

A controversial idea supported by Galileo Galilei in the 1600s was that the earth was not the center of the universe. This idea was prohibited by the Catholic Church for lack of empirical proof, and Galileo spent the last years of his life under house arrest because of this unconventional idea; he was only formally pardoned in 1992![6] Today, many unconventional minds offer alternative ideas and theories regarding health, cheap and clean energy sources, and the nature of humanity's existence. And even if those ideas are currently proven false by "experts," they go a long way to engage our intellect and raise our curiosity—and that might be a good thing for the development of new ideas, tools, and solutions.

Who knows—so-called alternative ideas may actually prove to be the truth, or at least give direction toward other truths. When humans first came up with the crazy ideas about giving man the ability to fly or one day walk on the moon, they were initially ridiculed; eventually, however, their ideas were accepted and became realities.

The following sampling of websites, books, and movies may inspire us to look at life differently and to open our minds to new approaches to sustainable HHP. They may also help us realize that we are more in control of our weaknesses of nature, our IMP, and our HHP than we are led to believe by outside forces.

- *What the Bleep.* This docudrama uses a great story, philosophical discussion, quantum physics, and visual science to theorize on such ideas as how our repeated thought patterns create neural pathways of habits and therefore create our reality. Testimonials abound from people who have immediately changed their lives for the better after watching this movie.

- *The Secret.* Though this movie also delves into the idea of thoughts creating reality, it focuses more on the law of attraction—the concept that our thoughts and feelings, especially passionate feelings, are largely responsible for attracting real events and things into our lives. Whether the law of attraction is real or not, this is truly a motivating movie.

- *Zeitgeist: The Movie.* This controversial movie, which is available for viewing online at zeitgeistmovie.com, offers a fascinating view at how the beliefs, agendas, desires, and dogmas of outside influences have been and are still controlling the way we think and act. It connects many religions through their common histories of celestial, sun, and earth worship. It also looks at how government and global economics are outdated and may have hidden agendas. True or not, the movie is of great interest to those who are trying to make sense of the current craziness in the world.

- *How To Eat, Move, and Be Healthy!* This book by Paul Chek is not a run-of-the-mill health and fitness book. It looks at the basics of how to get healthy, instead of how to avoid sickness, by explaining topics like food quality, exercise, energy systems, body toxins, digestion, pooping (Chek's word), sleep, and stress. Chek is sometimes looked at as a radical in the health and wellness field, but he is highly respected and gets amazing results with his clients, which include doctors, top athletes, and people for whom conventional methods have failed.

- *The No-Grain Diet.* A book by Dr. Joseph Mercola, who proposes that grains and sugars are the cause of many of the illnesses that plague the world today. For anyone serious about achieving optimal health, Dr. Mercola's book, along with his unconventional but informative website mercola.com, are a must.

- *A New Earth.* This book by Eckhart Tolle explores the human ego on many levels, including how the ego has a life of its own, feeds on inner and outer conflict, and distracts people and whole nations from the peaceful power of the present moment. Although some readers may consider the book "recycled Buddhism," it is nonetheless thought-provoking; at the very least, it gives us a look at why we suffer and then offers tools to break out of that suffering.

- *Power vs. Force: The Hidden Determinants of Human Behavior.* A book written by Dr. David Hawkins and appreciated by the likes of Lee Iacocca, Sam Walton, and Mother Teresa. Every page provokes and inspires the intellect, like the section that describes levels of human consciousness from the lowest negative forces of shame, guilt, fear, and anger (which interestingly represent a large part of the history of mankind) to the higher positive powers of willingness and acceptance (which our modern era has begun to touch), and then onward to the highest levels of love, joy, peace, and enlightenment where you find the likes of Jesus, Buddha, and Mohammed—a level that is likely the next step of our evolution.

- *Magical Child.* This book by Joseph Chilton Pearce is an intriguing, almost mystical, child-raising resource

> ### *Sun "Worship"?*
>
> *In the past, those who worshiped anything outside of accepted religious beliefs (such as the sun) were often labeled as heretics and treated with ridicule, fear, and violence. In this current day and age, it would be nice to think that we as a "civilized" society have matured to a point where we can safely worship both the ideologies and gods of our religions and, at the same time, one of nature's major components—our common star, the sun.*
>
> *Have you ever looked at the early-morning sun through squinted eyes? If you do so, you will see the glowing sun at the center of a distinct cross. (Be careful, though! Do not look directly, open the eyelids just a tiny fraction and only look for a split second.) A short, thick line rises directly up from the sun, two shorter thick lines run outwards from both sides, and one long, thick, glowing line runs straight down. Between these four distinct lines, numerous thinner lines radiate outwards.*
>
> *This "sun cross" is a symbolic figure in many religions, although it may have different origins and meanings in each one. Perhaps the symbol of the cross first came into being when cavemen recorded what they saw as they glanced at and worshipped the life-and-warmth-giving sun with squinted eyes.*
>
> *Are we on the cusp of a blessed era of constructive consciousness when all people can, in addition to any other beliefs, freely "worship" the sun as the life-giving body that it is?*

tool that gives insight as to what the natural billion-year-old biological unfolding/development of a child was meant to be. Pearce demonstrates beautifully that allowing a child the primary processes such as play, exploration, imagination, and experimentation (under the watchful eye of a parent), not the strictly programmed routines that our modern western society advocates, are essential in supporting the healthy balanced growth of a human being. A must-read for parents and those searching for answers to their own behaviors.

- *EnlightenNext®* magazine. A thought-provoking magazine (and website) with an East meets West dialogue of various perspectives on religion, spirituality, academics, and culture. It also explores the nature of reality, why we are here, and what's next in our evolution.

- *Humanity Ascending* (documentary series). An enlightening look at how humans are on the cusp of either entering into an era of global destruction or, by a process of necessity and survival, evolving with a quantum leap into something totally different but of immense beauty, much like a caterpillar transforms miraculously into a butterfly.

- *And more.* See HealthyIsm.com for more inspirational websites, books, and movies.

All humanity's great inventions and creations have come either from necessity or out-of-the-box imagination and pondering. Consider looking into these and other unconventional resources for inspiration and insight into your quest to welcome becoming an optimally healthy, enduringly happy, and peacefully prosperous human being.

On Our Way

We are on our way; HealthyIsm is possible! As we begin to calmly and kindly do what it takes to stop our destructive ways we lay the foundation for welcoming sustainable HHP into our lives and others.

The next section for consideration will go into more detail on how to overcome your Unhealthyolic behaviors, become a HealthyIst, and take control of your health by developing further an awareness of a few important points:

- Our lives are directed by our instincts and IMP.

- We, not someone else, are ultimately in control of our own lives.

- As a society we are maturing and waking up to the illusions around us. We are becoming "dis-illusioned."

- As a society, we are recognizing that we are more connected to each other and to the earth than we could ever have imagined.

- Many people, but currently still a small fraction of the world's population, are already awake and in control and willingly helping others achieve a healthy, constructive life.

The section will also offer a seven-step process that will lead you all the way to a life of HealthyIsm. The most important step is the first, which is exploring why we humans do such unhealthy things to ourselves, to others, to animals, and to our great earth.

CONSIDERATION II

Seven Steps to HealthyIsm

This second Consideration asks you to consider using a seven-step process to welcome a completely constructive lifestyle. Approach each step as part of a stairway ascending to higher and dryer ground, away from the tide of destructive illusions, instincts, and inner beliefs we now hold true.

These steps can be powerful, so be careful! If you are of sound mind and not suffering from mental problems, but you think you may have difficulty handling change or your emotions, ask a trusted, open-minded friend to be with you during the process. Or you can contact The HealthyIsm Organization through our website, and we'll connect you with someone who has already successfully completed the steps. If you think any part of this process is just too much for you, seek the help of a professionally recognized therapist.

Please note that for the following to be the most effective, you must be ready and willing to fully participate in your own "change for the better."

Step 1: What Happened to Us?

Humans are creatures of habit. Like any other animal, we follow a predictable daily routine. But unlike animals, we have the ability to self-reflect and look at our habits as constructive, neutral, or destructive.
—Gary Drisdelle, *HealthyIsm*

The more severe the pain or illness, the more severe will be the necessary changes. These may involve breaking bad habits or acquiring some new and better ones.
—Peter McWilliams, *Life 101*

Man has been endowed with reason, with the power to create, so that he can add to what he's been given. But up to now he hasn't been a creator, only a destroyer.
—Anton Chekhov, *Uncle Vanya*

What happened to us? How did we become so unhealthy and destructive to ourselves, others, and the world? Why do we do damaging things to our bodies and minds that we know are not good for us or for others? And what about the things that we *don't know* that cause us a life of pain and misery and a general lack of good HHP? By answering these questions and becoming aware of the origins of our destructiveness we begin the first step to welcoming a healthy I and a healthy world.

Root Causes of Our Unhealthyolic Lifestyles

If a car engine does not start a mechanic will look for the root cause(s) of the problem, such as a dead battery, faulty electronics, or an empty gas tank. Once the root cause is identified, then begins the fixing process.

The root causes of our Unhealthyolic lifestyles are brought about by two reasons—a lack of awareness of and weak control over our destructive instincts; and a lack of awareness of and weak control over our nurtured/programmed minds.

First, let's focus on our nurtured minds. Think about this: if "healthy" newborn babies from any corner of the globe—be it from neighboring, warring cultures or countries or from opposing religions—were raised together in an environment that allowed them to develop without hindrance or dysfunction from childhood to adulthood, and if they were free to explore and play, lovingly educated, taught to respect each other's backgrounds, taught about destructive instincts and inner mental programming and how to control them, kept free of a toxic environment, and provided with clean, nutritious food, the eventual result would undoubtedly be mature, rational adults who choose healthy, constructive lifestyles and live harmoniously with nature and each other.

As it stands, however, we are not raised in such a pristine, optimal environment. Our environment is toxic, our food is processed to death, and our minds are injured with archaic dogma. Our intake and assimilation of the thoughts and beliefs of others can set us up for destructiveness and feeling lost from the very beginning. As early as the age of four we leave the innocence of our *in-the-moment* nature self (play, explore, and laugh) and move into our *be-something-else* nurtured self (such as "sit still, leave that alone, do what I say, be like this, don't trust that skin color or culture" and "be serious!").

> ### Healthy I, Healthy Child
>
> "The apple doesn't fall far from the tree." Children are mostly a reflection of the parents they "fell" from. To change the apple, change the tree:
> - Be the human being you'd like them to be.
> - Have the same amount of patience with them as you'd like them to have with others.
> - Teach them about their destructive instincts and IMP.
> - Encourage them, but don't force them, to be aware of what an HHP choice is, even if they still choose otherwise.
> - It's okay if they don't heed you, because they are still hearing you.
> - Above all, remember the words of wisdom you received from your elders that you did not really "get" or accept until years later.
>
> Plant the seed, practice a constructive life and you will bear the fruit of healthy, happy and prosperous children.

The nurtured self, the inner mental programming conditioned into us from the time we are born, is a biggie when it comes to our destructive ways. We are taught early on by authority figures to think and act a certain way, and we continue to obediently "follow the program" merely because our parents told us to or someone who labeled himself an authority told us that he knows what's best for us. How often do you see commercials on TV that use an authority figure, like a gal in a white lab coat with a stethoscope or a guy smartly dressed in a suit, to sell a product? It happens all the time.

Milgram Experiment

For example, many people, through social conditioning, are taught to believe that only a doctor knows best, so when it comes to questions of health, they refuse to listen or be open to anyone or anything else. For some science on this phenomenon, read about the fascinating Milgram Experiment.[7] Originally conducted by Yale University psychologist Stanley Milgram in the 1960s, and replicated in 2006 by Santa Clara University professor Jerry Burger, the experiment showed that people will generally obey an authority figure (in this case, by giving supposedly very painful electric shocks to another person) to the point of executing acts that conflict with their personal conscience.

Because of social conditioning, we tend to do "everything" in a prescribed way, including the way we deliver babies. In his book *Magical Child,* Joseph Pearce shows how we are removed from the natural, healthy birth and growth that the universal biological process intended for us. He tells us that this disassociation starts from the moment of conception when many mothers are stressed and anxious and only become more so during the pregnancy and on into the busy delivery room, which in turn stresses the innocent baby.[8]

Pearce goes on to state that women have been having babies naturally since time began and most would do better without the routine that happens in most hospitals around the world today. If mothers lived healthy positive lives – if they lived in the moment of the beautiful miracle happening inside instead of in the anxiety of past problems and future fears—most childbirths would be amazing physical and emotional experiences, and most babies would be born without complication.

In effect, women could literally go into the woods, squat down, and have the baby on their own as nature intended, as millions have done in the past. In no way is it suggested that women do this, because there are plenty of advantages to having a safe, clean environment with a professional ready for the rare emergency. But by being aware of our programmed fearful perception of childbirth we can at least look at it as a mostly safe, natural, beautiful experience, and as the most important point at which a human life can begin optimal development.

Kyle's Home Birth

Our youngest son was born at home, and it was one of the most beautiful experiences of our lives. In retrospect, being fully involved in my other son Justyn's birth at the hospital was just as moving and wonderful. But there is something extra special about being in your own home, your castle, your place of love, with the other children sleeping peacefully in the next room.

When it was time, my amazing partner, Lekha, just calmly said it was so, and we called the midwives. Except for the moments when she had contractions, Lekha just continued with what she'd been doing, which was preparing eggplant parmesan. Only when we knew the moment was getting close did we move into the bedroom to await nature's process. With Lekha squatting (which is the way nature intended it, not lying on the back) and the lights dimmed, I was allowed the honor of guiding and catching our new baby boy Kyle as he entered this world. There was no bum-slapping, no poking and prodding, no worry about the baby breathing immediately (the umbilical cord, still attached, has up to 10 minutes of nutrients, including "air supply").[9] Kyle went directly from birth to Mom; then they both rested for at least five minutes before we clamped the cord. Then off to bed for both to catch some rest, but not before Lekha asked me to feed the midwives.

Lekha was up and about the very next day with no complications. A truly beautiful in-the-now experience for all involved. Kyle today, at age six, is the most beautiful, joyful, and busy boy who never gets sick and always wants to play and explore.

IMP (Inner Mental Programming): The Little Troublemaker Within

Let's look further at the little troublemaker within our heads that allows our lives to be ruled by habit-producing thoughts and beliefs—our inner mental programming.

Your IMP is a personal collection of beliefs and values that acts like a computer software program that dictates the way you act, think, and move through life. Many people don't realize that we are submerged in this mentally programmed-driven culture any more than a fish realizes that it's swimming in water. It is basically an unconscious driver behind all the things you think and do…unconscious until now, that is. Hello, IMP! (Yes, the IMP in your head!)

Your IMP is formed through the varied experiences and sensory input (what you take in through your five main senses and other special senses as shown in the following grey area) that you receive throughout your life, all of which ultimately program your mind and influence your perception of reality.

On the immediate personal level, your view of reality is formed largely by the information conveyed to you by your parents, upbringing (cultural, religious, and political influences), and community (rich or poor); generational influences; peers and mentors; authority figures (like lawyers, doctors, and "experts"); and your elders.

On a more global societal level, your beliefs and perceptions are influenced by media and news programs; advertising; megacorporations that tell us what foods to eat, what products to buy,

Your Five Senses (And Counting!)

Your IMP is created by the input of information from the world around you through the obvious sensors of the human body that you learned about in school:
1. taste
2. touch
3. smell
4. sight
5. hearing

We also talk of other senses that may or may not be a blend of the above senses. These senses also provide us with information:
1. time of day
2. direction; magnetoception (or magnetorecption)
3. proprioception, or sense of position to self (e.g., where your hand is in relation to your head) and sense of the world and objects around you
4. hunger; fullness
5. thermoception (sense of temperature)
6. pain
7. being "in the zone" or "in the now"
8. balance
9. deceleration and acceleration
10. isolation
11. humor
12. memory
13. feeling well or content
14. full bladder
15. fashion and color
16. belonging

Your Five Senses (And Counting!), continued

We can also add psychic senses into the mix, such as the sense of:
1. intuition (the ability to know what to do without reasoning)
2. premonition (the sense that something is going to happen)
3. déjà vu (the sense you've experienced a new situation before)
4. being watched
5. peace and safety
6. danger
7. enlightenment
8. whether someone is telling the truth or lying
9. consciousness
10. oneness or connectivity (which may be "in-the-zone-ness")[10,11]

Having a "sense" of the multitude of ways that we receive information from the world around us will help us in our quest to recognize our weaknesses and welcome in a life of HealthyIsm.

and how to live; governments (which are highly influenced by the mega-corporations); and schools (which are largely regulated by government).

Every one of those elements conveys its system of belief and perception, both beneficial and destructive, onto you.

Your life, then, depends on what you do with the belief/perception system, the inner mental programming that's been your guidance since birth.

A large amount of this guidance was positive or provided a foundation to further development, like don't touch the fire or eating an apple a day or knowing that $E=mc^2$ or investing wisely or making it a point to follow the Golden Rule.

But some of the other "stuff" just bogged you down, took the control of your own destiny out of your hands, and led you into unconscious bad habits and unhealthy lifestyles: stuff like thinking you must eat according to subjectively developed food guides, or adapt behaviors as defined by "family" TV shows, or shop till you drop to consume many more products than you need, or cause pain and trouble to others as a result of one perception of an ancient ideology.

By being shown by others (who were also submersed in their own programming) how to think, you operated in life like the unsuspecting, easy target of a stage hypnotist. You've been seductively hypnotized by all the illusions in your environment and in your head.

Remember that the term "illusion" doesn't mean to say

that something doesn't exist. Rather, an illusion in this sense is something that creates a barrier between our pure essence—of our own flesh and bones, heartbeat, and breath—and the pure essence of the rest of nature, such as plants, animals, babies, and the living planet. We need to become aware of our interconnection with all of this.

Consider the breakdown of the different types of illusions and realities:

- **Outer illusions** include anything manmade, like television, time/clocks, cars, and nutrition guides. Each of these things may have great benefits, but if what you see on television dominates your sense of reality, if you are a slave to time, if a sense of anonymity and separation causes you to drive without heeding the safety of others, and if you blindly follow a food guide without also observing the effects on your own health, then the use of these illusions are ultimately destructive to self and others.
- **Outer realities** include anything untouched by man, like forests, oceans, wild animals, witnessing the love between a child and mother or between other human beings, the earth below, the universe above, and everything natural in between.
- **Inner illusions** include your belief system, the busy babble constantly streaming in your head, and your programmed perception of the world around you.
- **Inner realities** include your heartbeat, breathing, non-thoughts, awareness of oneness, being "in the zone," peacefulness, love, smiling for no reason, engaging with nature, such as simply holding hands with your child (one of nature's finest and most beautiful creations).

The illusions and realities around you are co-programmers of the belief systems in your head—the IMP—which, in turn, either promote a constructive, healthy life or a destructive, unhealthy one.

Your *destructive* IMP whines along on the surface—I want this, I want that, I want to make this destructive choice—and wants to be "kept busy" with continuous indulgence (at least it thinks it wants that). An unaware nature self will be ruled by its IMP.

On the other hand, your constructive IMP supports an optimal evolution and searches for the best ways for your human life form to survive. Your true nature self—your animal body—wants to be healthy. It belongs to no one, not even your IMP—and if it did "belong" to someone, it would belong to God, Universal Spirit, the evolutionary pulse, or whatever force that makes electrons orbit the nucleus, planets orbit the sun, babies grow, and flowers bloom. This force meant and intended for your body to live and die healthfully and to be treated well; it also meant for your being to live in harmony with the earth and its inhabitants.

The lack of control you have over your IMP is the granddaddy of all the reasons for your destructive habits. Think of it as the umbrella under which many of the other reasons presented in this chapter take shelter.

If you want to know what your IMP has been up to, just take a look at your life, at the current condition of your HHP. If you are unhappy and have an unhealthy body, unhealthy relationships, and a life of scarcity, it's safe to place most of the blame on the destructive side of your IMP.

Your Personal IMP Is Like a Folklore Imp

In folklore, an imp is a small, mischievous creature who goes around causing trouble but who, nonetheless, has the ability to do good. Your personal IMP is somewhat the same. Depending on how (and if) you control it, it can cause you trouble or do you good. It's the nurtured mindset that largely dictates, or at least tries to dictate, what you think, what actions you take, and ultimately what will become of your life. The idea is to keep the belief systems and programming that empower you and help you live a healthy, happy, and prosperous life and to control or stop the ones who keep you stuck in destructive habits.

For many people, just the act of recognizing this mischievous IMP for what it is would be enough to propel them into great HHP. When you can name the problem, you are well on your way to solving that problem. Your IMP controls your thoughts and, therefore, your life; being aware of and taming your IMP is a huge part of the solution!

Your thoughts can either evolve you or destroy you. The fact that many people (perhaps from seeing so much misery in the news) believe humanity is on the brink of complete destruction and are thinking and acting destructively is a direct result of some of those past and current programmed thoughts.

The good news is that there is a growing percentage of people (as witnessed by the popularity of alternative evolutionary thinkers like Eckhart Tolle, Andrew Cohen, Deepak Chopra, James Redfield, Neal Donald Walsh, and Barbara Marx Hubbard) who believe we are evolving in the direction of awareness of our IMP, and who are glimpsing an essence of oneness, of the interconnectivity that may bring peace, love, enlightenment, and human ascendance.

How can we, as human beings, assist in the positive evolution of ourselves and the planet? How can we transcend our old destructive values that are causing many people a life of disease, sadness, and deficiency? By relentlessly practicing awareness of the IMP that controls us, stopping destructive habits, and welcoming a healthy I.

What Were We Thinking?

Here's an example of how IMP has done us harm:

Most people would accept that a mother's bonding with her child is extremely important to the child's development. But thanks to some propaganda in the 1950s, mothers were discouraged from kissing and holding their babies too much because it was believed to be a bad thing.[12] Do you think this may have contributed to some dysfunction in our society?

Destructive Instincts

Married to the IMP, the grand-daddy of the origin of your destructive habits, is the grand-mommy: your instincts. Whatever they're called—be it unconscious urges, mammalian behavior, inclinations, compulsions, tendencies, propensities, or instincts—sometimes we feel or do things that we were not taught or shown, things that at one point helped us survive and evolve as a species.

Many of these instincts are beautiful! The primal instincts to care for our children, to work together for the common good, to gather food, to share, to play, to create artistically and mechanically, to create tools for better or more secure living, to communicate with others, to adapt to the situation at hand, to be curious, explore, and seek answers to questions, and to laugh and find humor in our daily lives are all great and must be nurtured.[13]

But sometimes humans take actions that aren't so great, actions that are the result of unleashed urges that cause us to do harmful things to self, others, or the earth. Is it possible that many instincts that were once strengths in our evolution and had a survival purpose are now sometimes unnecessarily acted upon, causing destruction and contributing to much chaos in people's lives and in the world?

Absolutely! When we lived off the land, roamed as tribes, and hunted and gathered with our bare hands, thriving as predators and scavengers, we relied on hidden urges and the resulting cascade of emotions to guide our actions. Consider some of the human instincts that kept our predecessors alive, for example: fight, flight, or freeze; hunt or hide; gather and hoard; mating;

and joining others to make strong tribes. Greed and hoarding for one's self or one's clan made a lot of sense when it was a way to ensure the survival of one's tribe. We knew that another's gain was our loss and vice versa. But in the present day, acquiring more than one's family could use in a lifetime—or even two or three lifetimes—while not doing enough to help others acquire, maintain, and go beyond their own basic needs is totally unnecessary and ultimately destructive to the world and to ourselves. Once a person is abundantly comfortable, it makes sense to offer the tools, resources, and education to others so that they are at least able to comfortably provide the basic necessities for themselves.

It's not easy to recognize and control destructive instincts, especially since much of our modern world accepts them as natural; thus we operate in a fearful, animalistic survival mode much like the alpha male instinct in which there is one winner and a bunch of losers. We *naturally* teach our children to compete with each other, to understand that there is always a winner and a loser—just think of children's games like musical chairs. Then those children grow up and push others away so they can get one of the limited chairs of privileges like abundant or excessive food, water, land, money, comfort, and other resources.

The list of "instincts" in the following chart is meant to help us recognize that some of what we do or feel may be the result of hidden urges. This is not a complete list; it is merely an illustration of how certain destructive behaviors can be attributed to important evolutionary survival instincts that have often caused, and continue to cause, havoc in our lives and in our world.

Instinct	How It Helped Our Evolution	How It Can Hurt Us Now
Jealousy Instinct (the release of hostile hormones/how we react when people we love or lust for are approached by someone else)	By keeping others away from one's mate, one was also protecting the chance of passing on one's gene pool.	Untamed jealousy causes foggy thinking, aggressive behavior, and unnecessary strife in many situations and relationships.
Envy Instinct (wanting what someone else has)	Wanting and getting what someone else had was often a matter of life or death and had to be acted upon.	Envy often causes stress and depression through the perpetual comparison of what we have versus what "they" have (the must-keep-up-with-the-Joneses cycle).
Mating Instinct	Caveman saw cavewoman, his sexual hormones started racing, and he set out to have cavewoman and produce offspring.	In today's civilized world, most men and woman control their sexual urges. But there are still those people who are overcome with instinctual hormones and act strangely—and possibly dangerously—toward others instead of using intellect and non-aggressive courting rituals.

Instinct	How It Helped Our Evolution	How It Can Hurt Us Now
Greed/Hoarding Instinct (acquiring as much as possible for oneself and one's family)	Having access to a store of goods ensured survival of self and offspring in times of famine.	Individuals, families, and countries still gather/hoard resources for their "own kind" to ensure long-term survival. It is a difficult circumstance in our modern world as populations grow and the earth's resources decline.
"Ridiculing Others" Instinct (building oneself up by putting others down)	This was perhaps a means of compensating for or masking one's own weaknesses.	Today we call this a form of bullying that can result in the low self-esteem and sense of worthlessness or powerlessness in others.
"Need to Be Right" Instinct (inability to accept that what we say or do is incorrect)	Having flawed judgment or knowledge often meant trouble or death.	Even when we know we are wrong, many of us will lie or rigorously defend our positions. This behavior leads to stressful situations like road rage or clashing cultures.
"Making Things Simpler and Easier" Instinct	Nature loves efficiency, and humans instinctually aim for simpler, easier, and more efficient lives.	In some ways, humans have made things so efficient or simple that we've ended up not having to use our minds or bodies (think of using a calculator or a moving sidewalk), which contributes to weaker minds and bodies.

Instinct	How It Helped Our Evolution	How It Can Hurt Us Now
Anger and Aggression Instinct (self-protection)	When caught in a corner or surrounded by attackers, the instinct to display frightful characteristics helped one's chances of surviving the attack.	When people are confronted about something they did or said they often react by blaming others or with verbal or physical aggression. Today, whole nations threatened by neighboring countries over issues of land, religion, or politics retaliate with military aggression.
Fear Instinct (distress aroused by impending danger)	Keeping constant, fearful vigilance for potential threats to oneself or the tribe bettered the chances of preparing for or reacting to an attack.	Many people live in constant fear of what could happen, thereby cheating themselves out of the beauty of the present moment or a hopeful future.
Laziness Instinct (resistance to work or any exertion)	Conserving energy or being "lazy," like lions in the midday sun, helped one's chance of survival by saving that energy for when it was most needed, such as gathering food, hunting, or running from being hunted.	Some individuals are permanent "lazy lions" that have little drive or energy and therefore have a hard time making an effort to accomplish anything, whether it be exercising, eating properly, improving education, creating abundance in their lives, or otherwise "gathering" a stable, constructive life.

Instinct	How It Helped Our Evolution	How It Can Hurt Us Now
Alpha Male Instinct (the urge to dominate or be better than others in a group)	Having one dominant leader that rose to the top in a group brought order and helped the tribe achieve a stronger position over its environment and competing groups. This, in turn, improved the group's ability to survive.	Some people today, especially males, have the urge to outdo another's talent, ability, or performance. He might feel threatened by another's position of power and use aggressive or manipulative behaviors to prove his own worth and better his own position. Alpha male hierarchies in cultures, social status, and corporate structure give the biggest piece of pie to a few while the masses share a tiny piece.
Gossip Instinct (talking about others regarding their behavior, status, appearance, etc.)	In the past, learning as much as possible about those around you, such as a potential mate or a potential foe, was linked to a better chance of survival and the passing on of our genetic pool.[14]	Today, gossip can still be beneficial when used to spread good news or keep tabs on people in our lives. But often gossip is destructive and a form of bullying.

Instinct	How It Helped Our Evolution	How It Can Hurt Us Now
"Distrusting People 'Not Like Us'" Instinct	People felt safer living in groups with others who shared the same religion, culture, perception of reality, ideology, traits, manners, and customs, and who they knew to be stable, trustworthy, and reliable (as opposed to strangers from whom they didn't know what to expect.	Distrusting or disliking "quirky" people or people who are different from us causes needless and destructive separation between humans.
"Blending in With the Crowd" Instinct	Keeping a low profile (like not making eye contact) meant less chance to be singled out and harmed by the alpha male or others wishing to prove that they were the stronger alpha.	Today, many people don't make contact or get involved in activities in which they can excel and be noticed for fear that their conspicuous position might attract harmful actions or judgment from others

There are many other destructive behaviors that are rooted in survival skills, such as the crying instinct (used to get attention to satisfy one's needs), the territorial instinct (used to claim and dominate a land), and the war instinct (used to destroy a threat to one's tribe).

Practicing HealthyIsm does not mean ignoring or turning off our instincts; it simply means *recognizing* any destructive instinctual drives and controlling them. In fact, there may be times when we need to give in to our urges. If we actually come face to face with an angry, protective mama bear or a mugger on the street, then we must go with our instincts and either fight, flee, or freeze. But if we are cut off in traffic or someone unfairly jumps in front of us in line—because that person is succumbing to his/her own weak control—we must recognize and control our brute animalistic urge to compete or retaliate, defend ourselves, and survive, and instead use the more highly evolved, methodic, conscious part of the human brain, the cortex, to think first and do something constructive next—such as practicing calmness and focusing on the breath, counting to 10, and letting the other person "get away with it." In many situations, not retaliating is usually our best choice because one of three things typically happens in any confrontation: we get hurt, they get hurt, we all get hurt—and none of these outcomes are good.

Destructive instincts cause havoc on an even larger scale, too. Painful world conflicts like culture clashes, religious quarrels, and land disputes can all be traced back to humans who acted with the instinctual, largely unconscious, reptilian part of their brains. It was, and still is, all about a fear of something. It's time to change that fear to a calm and kind awareness and welcome in peaceful resolutions.

Other Forces That Fuel Our Destructive Lifestyles

Our IMP and our instincts are the foundation of our destructive lifestyles and are also the basis of various other forces in our lives. As you read through the list below, think about your own life and how any of these forces may relate to you.

1. The Pleasure-Pain Principle

We innately seek pleasure and avoid pain; that is one explanation as to why some people exercise and some don't. People who exercise either take pleasure in the actual exercise or foresee pleasure in the outcome of a fit, healthy, good-looking body. People who don't exercise perhaps only feel the temporary pain of the actual exercise and never last long enough to see or feel the long-term pleasurable results. The pain of an uncomfortable life brought on by any reason (like poverty, abuse, or lack of knowledge) is often masked by a short-term pleasure such as using drugs or alcohol, commiserating with others, or eating junk food.

2. Lack of Knowledge or Awareness

If you don't know that something is harmful, and it feels good for the moment, there's a good chance you'll continue doing it. For example, if you don't know that the daily, pervasive, and excessive consumption of most grains, even the widely advertised "whole wheat," may cause many long-term physical problems, then obviously you will continue eating those grains. After all, how can you make a change if you aren't aware that a particular choice is causing your joint pain or digestive problems?

> ## *Pleasure and Pain*
>
> *Most of the things we do in our lives we do to either avoid pain or seek pleasure—in fact, research shows that this pain/pleasure equation is a basic human survival technique that dates back to our earliest ancestors. Our primal urge is to experience pleasure and steer clear of hurt. Think of the cavemen: when some action or behavior released good-feeling chemicals into the blood stream and inspired warm, pleasant feelings—be it intimacy, taking in the sun, or biting into a piece of sweet fruit—then they were naturally drawn toward that pleasure-giver again and again. Likewise, they learned to avoid what caused them pain—the yearning from lack of intimacy, a plant that made them ill, or too much sun that burned their skin.*
>
> *Genetically, we may still have a lot in common with the cavemen, but modern society has unfortunately (and inevitably) presented us with modern problems. While it's true that nowadays there is a plethora of instant pleasure-giving substances like sugary treats, chemically enhanced foods, alcohol, and legal and illegal drugs, it is equally true that many of them eventually damage our bodies, usually sooner than later. But our drive to seek pleasure is so strong that, although the logical mind may recognize the long-term unhealthy action, it will be completely overridden by the "pleasure now!" area of the mind—unless we learn to notice our primal urges and the resulting desires and to take control of them.*

3. Physical Dependence

Some of your habits may be labeled as physical dependence

and, in certain cases, you may need professional guidance to overcome them and receive treatment for the withdrawal symptoms. When you stop those habits, your body goes through a withdrawal period that causes a state of "dysphoria" (opposite of euphoria). However, authors like Allen Carr, who delves into the subject in his bestselling book *The Easy Way to Stop Smoking,* say that the severity of withdrawal is largely dependent on your *beliefs* about stopping a habit.[15] And where do those beliefs come from? That's right—from your IMP!

4. Psychological Addiction

To paraphrase Dr. Avram Goldstein, a professor of pharmacology at Stanford University, an addiction occurs when a person establishes a regular pattern of use of a substance, which then becomes more important than "normal," healthy activities. This is the disease model which says that addictive behavior is "the business of the brain" and that the user has no control. The other side of the story, as shown in the Rat Park experiment conducted by Canadian psychologist Bruce K. Alexander, is that when a rat is given a choice of drugged water or non-drugged water in pleasant liv-

> **Filling a Void**
>
> *Many humans who do unhealthy things to their lives are unconsciously or consciously trying to fill a void. A lonely or sad person may overeat or drug himself because he is missing love. A person who has used a drug once—and as a result was able to escape all sense of time and space and feel euphoric, connected to Nature, Universal Spirit, or to God because of it—may very likely do it again and again because he misses those feelings and experiences.*

ing conditions, there will be no addiction—and that may indicate that your environment largely influences your choices and desires.[16]

5. Lack of Constructive Guidance or Mentors

If you have no mentor to help get you and keep you on the right path, you may needlessly strike out many times on your own. Take care, however, to do your research to ensure that you are guided by a trustworthy mentor or reputable information. You can consider this book and the HealthyIsm organization itself as your mentor…after you do your research on us!

6. Presence of Destructive Guidance or Mentors

The information and "guidance" you receive from individuals, institutions, and the media is not always in your best interest. Surrounding yourself with people who have similar unhealthy or destructive habits is simply a means of gaining support and justification for those habits.

7. Follow-the-Herd Mentality

In addition to being guided by your friends, you are also often guided by the herd, or "groupthink." Groupthink is the phenomenon of doing whatever society dictates—without analyzing and evaluating ideas for yourself—for fear of upsetting society, being seen as an outsider, or being downright ostracized.

8. Lack of Vision or Clear, Constructive Goals

Living without clear, constructive goals for all areas of your life is like traveling without a map—you have less of a chance of arriving at your destination safe and sound!

9. Limited Choices Due to Environmental Factors

For some people, factors like poverty, lack of access to needed supplies, corrupt governments, oppressive regimes, and toxic environments limit the choices and opportunities for achieving healthy, happy, and prosperous lives.

10. Too Many Choices

On the other hand, people who live reasonably well-off lives in a stable country often act like kids in a candy store. Because they have easy access to fleeting-pleasure stuff like junk food, alcohol, drugs, and even escalators instead of stairs, they tend to go for instant gratification, which brings gradual suffering.

> **Another Example of IMP Control**
>
> *Based on some flawed studies in the 1950s, the "experts," and then the public, accepted the idea that all fat was bad for you. Among other things, we were told that fat caused heart disease and made us fat—and we all bought it. We became obsessed with low-fat this and low-fat that. Only now, half a century later, have we begun to recognize that certain fats are not only good for you, they are actually essential to many bodily functions like the building of cell membranes and the production of various hormones.*[17,18]

11. The Snowball Effect

Submersion in an unhealthy lifestyle creates a vicious momentum. People caught in a cycle of unhealthy habits often think thoughts like, "Oh, I'm already unhealthy, so why don't I give in and have that unhealthy thing," and "There's no hope for me anyway"—thoughts that eventually become self-fulfilling prophecies.

12. The "Why Bother?" Effect: Witnessing a "Healthy" Person Become Unhealthy

Sometimes a person's reasons for being an Unhealthyolic stem from seeing close friends or family suffer from a devastating disease and die young even though that loved one had practiced a "healthy" lifestyle. Such an experience may lead the person into a *Why bother?* attitude in which he thinks, "You see? I may as well go crazy and have fun." If you are one of those people, your view of "quality vs. quantity" may feel right or even be "correct." But perhaps new reasoning formed by reading the information provided in this book or elsewhere—along with your intuitive feelings—will eventually lead you to a different conclusion. Perhaps you'll look at the situation from another angle: that because the afflicted person had led a healthy lifestyle, he may have actually improved his life expectancy by many years, even though he died young. Or that even though the person didn't smoke or drink, his so-called "healthy" diet may actually have been wreaking havoc on his system such as consuming only low-fat foods.

Overcoming Follow-the-Herd Mentality

Because we are controlled by our IMP, we are often shamed, chastised, or ridiculed if we don't follow the prescribed ideas of our society (the notion that war is necessary if it's for the *right* reasons), a particular religion (live this way or you'll not be accepted), the media (eat your fortified "food" to be healthy), or our parents (do as I say because I was raised this way).

That we willingly take certain actions that are detrimental to our health and to the health of our planet can be partly attributed to a phenomenon called "follow-the-herd mentality." Through his studies, American psychologist Solomon E. Asch showed that many people are apt to follow group opinion and succumb to social pressure *even if it means doing or saying something that is obviously incorrect.* Only a small, select group of people will think and act outside of group opinion.[19]

Historically, new ideas, systems, and procedures presented to the public are often met first with ridicule and skepticism, then with anger, and then eventually with widespread acceptance. *I know there are those who question* the validity of the works of some of the authors and creative thinkers who are mentioned in this book; that is fine and to be expected. At the same time, in order to take control of our lives, we must allow all people to explore (without ridicule or anger) their own and others' ideas, proven or unproven—for in doing so we open our own minds to new and thought-provoking possibilities. We need only remember that, though the Luddites at the turn of the nineteenth century resisted the changes brought on by the Industrial Revolution, those changes eventually became commonplace. This book, too, contains a few ideas that are still being ridiculed by mainstream society—and it encourages you not to be a Luddite, but rather to consider these ideas, and find the ones that will help you to welcome improved health, happiness, and prosperity. It encourages you to dedicate your *life* to finding out what works best for *you* and, ultimately, the world.

What Is a Habit?

What things do you do regularly and, usually, subconsciously?
- *Did you read the last page of this book first?*
- *Do you have coffee and something sweet every morning?*
- *Do you brush your teeth daily?*
- *Do you smoke a cigarette after every meal?*
- *Do you race cars that pass you on the highway?*
- *Do you take a daily walk?*

A habit, good or bad, is formed by repeating an action or behavior enough times that a neural pathway is created in the brain, much like regularly walking the same way in a field will create a distinct path in the earth. To change a bad habit, you have to stop doing it for an extended period of time, which will allow the pathway to "grow over." Then it's time to blaze new trails of constructive habits.

Repeated Actions Become Habits

Whatever the reason for our Unhealthyolic behaviors, once we repeat an action over and over again, we re-enforce the pattern and unconsciously create a habit. Habits are really just repeated thoughts and actions, and many of those thoughts are shaped and conditioned by the society in which we live. Western society, for example, has created a habit of eating certain meals at particular times of the day—breakfast means cereal, bagel, and coffee in the morning; lunch means a sandwich with processed meat and condiments at noon; dinner means grabbing some fast food on the way home in the evening. We have also created a dog-eat-dog economic system that panders to the elite and exploits the poor. Like Pavlov's dog, we have learned to salivate when the bell rings. And in the process of letting ourselves be conditioned, we have moved away from understanding our own personal constructive-life-formula and observing what works best for humanity.

We are largely unconscious of most of our unhealthy actions. Indeed, we may actually believe that we are doing well for ourselves because we have left the state of our health and lives in the hands of others, instead of being our own best health expert, nutritionist, and exercise trainer. All the programmers of your life—parents, culture, schools, media, peers—greatly influence the unhealthy way you think and act.

As a result of all those influences that become our IMP, coupled with destructive instincts, the majority of humans are like the proverbial lab rats taught to follow the path in the maze in a certain way and sequence, all for the little kernel of self-comfort and social acceptance we'll find tossed in a forgotten corner.

We have given into these self-comfort illusions that have become irresistible, cravings for things we *think* we need: conspicuous shopping; sugar in every form from candy, soda, and ice cream to breads, sauces, and processed meats; and hours of mindless television and video games. And the fun continues as we not only over-consume things that are negative for our lives but also over-consume products that are negative for everyone and everything else around us. As research analyst Victor Lebow said in 1950, "Our

> *The goal of life is living in agreement with nature.*
> —Zeno (335–264 BC)
> *from Diogenes Laertius, Lives of Eminent Philosphers*

enormously productive economy demands that we make consumption our way of life…we seek spiritual satisfaction, our ego satisfaction, in consumption."[20] It's true—as we have been trained to do since we were young, we consume and consume and consume, buy things that we don't need or might use once (if at all), because we think it is the correct thing to do. But, instead, our consumption becomes a habit—an unending attempt to fill our hole of unhappiness, to satisfy our ego, and to make ourselves feel complete. In reference to the ego-ic mind, Eckhart Tolle points out in *A New Earth* that "…when those thought forms operate, no possession, place, person, or condition will ever satisfy you."[21]

Until we find and take control of the root of those thought forms, our habits will continue. And remember: HealthyIsm does not say you must stop all "destructive" behaviors (since they may add a little spice and fleeting moments of happiness to your life); what it does say is that we must be aware and in control of them.

Driving Madly By

I live in a wonderful country with many things to be grateful for, like a stable government, abundant resources, generally good weather, diverse cultural acceptance, access to education, and cradle-to-grave medical services. One would think there would be great happiness—but I see so much unhappiness and anger in people who are *lost in IMP thoughts* and instinctual behaviors, like those people with frowning faces in the supermarket and those others driving madly by, running stop signs and looking important (so they think) as they chat on their cell phones with someone else who is lost. People can't be blamed for their thoughts and actions, as most of them are unaware of their IMP and destructive instincts. They are programmed by the influences of their upbringing and continue to be programmed by thousands of advertisements per day that tell them how to act and consume. They are led around by their noses, blindly accepting everything they are told. In the process of indulging in all these illusions of happiness, we have neglected to embrace and engage in the present moment and all of nature's wonderful realities, like our heartbeats, our own vibrant bodies, plants and animals, the earth, the stars, other humans, and especially our children. Of course there are also many constructive illusions—tools and toys, buildings and bridges, computers and the Internet—that are good or fun or support us.

In fact, indulging in those illusions of happiness, those pursuits of joy and convenience, may actually be healthy to a certain extent—who can deny that an occasional spin on a merry-go-round can create memories of happiness for a child? But suppose the child never wanted to get off? Many adults never want to get off their merry-go-round life of indulgences like tasty junk food, constant cell phone usage, excessive merchandise consumption, alcohol, and drugs; they're always chasing that momentary good feeling. But watch and learn: eventually the child gets off the merry-go-round. We must do the same by limiting and controlling or, if needed, stopping our own indulgences.

Whose Fault Is It?

We know it makes sense not to raise a cat in a pool, because a cat's environment is earth and air, not water. Yet many of us humans are living out of our elements, splashing about in destructive instincts and murky "IMP water" that is not favorable to a constructive life.

Somehow, the beautiful frontal lobe of our brains which has given us the blessings of rational conscious thought and creative ability has, at the same time, cursed us with destructive thinking patterns.

If a person feels guilt, depression, anger, or any other negative emotion as a result of destructive thinking, there is some good news. It is possible to move beyond those emotions by knowing and accepting the fact that someone or something else likely messed up your thinking along the way. What does that mean?

It's not your fault!

Let's qualify that statement a bit: If you have been unaware of your destructive instincts and the IMP that has been controlling your every action, then it's not your fault that you practice an unhealthy lifestyle.

However, if you are now aware of your IMP—and yet you continue to do the same destructive things you're doing—then it's time to admit that you have some work to do. It's okay! Just follow the steps in the subsequent chapters and you'll be well on your way to controlling your destructive habits.

Destructive Nurture

NATURE-THOUGHTS/ACTIONS:
When a caveman was in need of food and saw fruit in a tree, his "natural instinctual thinking" would help him find the best method of obtaining it, such as climbing the tree. He did not need to be taught.

NURTURE-THOUGHTS/ACTIONS:
Eventually, that caveman showed his tribe members and nurtured his offspring on his best fruit-gathering techniques. Some nurture-thoughts were constructive—climb, poke the fruit with a stick, or build a ladder. Others were destructive—cut down the tree.

The challenge today is that people are being taught destructive methods of living their lives to get their fruits of comfort or conformity but end up cutting down the tree of a constructive life, so to speak.

It might be too much to expect a young or unaware person to change his ways, but there is no excuse for a mature, "aware," rational adult not to do the constructive thing. Do you find yourself conforming to destructive beliefs, over-consuming things you don't need, attacking someone if verbally provoked, making racial slurs, eating the same harmful diet that your parents consumed, or exploiting others because that's the way the system works?

If you do find that you are giving in to destructive nurture, then it's time to take control and climb, not cut down, the tree of a constructive life.

Bottom Line

At this point in our evolution, through constructive thinking and collaboration, all humans have the opportunity to be healthy, happy, and peacefully prosperous. We do not have to succumb to the weakness of character we see throughout the world today.

> ### *Negative Thoughts Spread Like Wildfire*
>
> *I was standing third in line at the library checkout counter with an armload of books and videos that I needed to research this book. What happened next was unbelievable. The two customers ahead of me at the only available checkout counter had the largest amount of stuff to check out that I have ever seen—in the range of 50 to 100 items each. I could feel my impatience rising, but I closed my eyes and meditated, focusing on my breath and the beauty of the now until I felt more relaxed. But I could feel and hear the agitation accumulating in the long line forming behind me. In an angry voice, one lady yelled, "Come on, open another teller!" Others fell right into the moment and started heckling the clerks. I looked around me and couldn't help thinking that all these people were asleep, that they had no idea that they were just falling into the same old programming. I kept thinking that I must intervene with a loving tone, affirm that this too shall pass—but I didn't. I just kept quiet. About 25 minutes later, I was finally able to check out my things. As I left the library, I could still feel the agitation and anger of the mob inside. Another lady was pulling her young son out the door, yelling very publicly and very embarrassingly at the boy. I felt so much for him and remember his mother saying, "You make me so angry..."*
>
> *We must take control of our minds, put things in perspective, and practice patience.*

We are the stewards of our world, externally and internally. We are meant to take care of our bodies as the temples that they are. We must take care of each other, our children, our environment, our dwelling home, and our earth home, as well as all things that inhabit it.

The actions we take for our own health affect everything else. We are all one. Even if a person doesn't believe that we are all connected in a quantum–holographic-ocean-of-oneness way, we can certainly all agree that we all breathe the same air and are an integral part of the same living (or dying?) planet.

It seems that many of us ignore or are unconscious of this possibility of oneness. We are so messed up by our lack of control over our nurture and nature that we are incapable of doing anything about it. Until now, that is, for if you are reading this, then you have entered an important step in creating a healthy I—knowing that you don't know! And the nice thing about that is that once you become aware of what's happening in your head and in the world around you, you can never again be fooled.

We need to take control of our IMPish minds and spend time cultivating good thoughts so we can healthily develop to a happy old age as nature intended.

A compelling reason to change; a growing awareness; gaining control over your IMP; understanding and managing your instincts; and throw in a little love and forgiveness—these are the elements that will provide you with the greatest chance of naturally releasing the underlying causes that made you develop your destructive lifestyle in the first place.

With all that in mind, it's time to discover what's going on in your current world. It's time to discover the truth and assess the damage, if there is any.

Step 1 Exercise: Discover the Underlying Destructive Forces of the World

Take a moment to look at the way things are in the world.

On this page, on a separate piece of paper, or on your computer, record any obvious destructive instincts and programmed behaviors that could be causing havoc in the world, such as the greed/hoarding instinct or harmful religious or parental inner mental programming. Your list may be a review of ideas expressed in this chapter, or perhaps you'll come up with some of your own ideas as to why we are so destructive.

_____

_____

_____

_____

_____

_____

_____

_____

_____

Step 2: What's Your Current Truth?

It is not the possession of truth, but the success which attends the seeking after it, that enriches the seeker and brings happiness to him.
—Max Planck

All truths are easy to understand once they are discovered; the point is to discover them.
—Galileo Galilei

"You have been telling the people that this is the Eleventh Hour, now you must go back and tell the people that this is the Hour. And there are things to be considered . . .
Where are you living?
What are you doing?
What are your relationships?
Are you in right relation?
Where is your water?
Know your garden.
It is time to speak your Truth.
Create your community.
Be good to each other.
And do not look outside yourself for the leader."
Then he clasped his hands together, smiled, and said,
"This could be a good time!"
—attributed to an unnamed Hopi elder
Hopi Nation, Oraibi, Arizona[22]

Now that you have the basis of why you do the destructive things that you do to yourself, to others, and to the earth, the next step is to take a snapshot of what your life is like right now. It's time to reveal the current truth of various aspects of your life.

Assess the Damage (If There Is Any)

When a tornado heads for a community, people rush into their basements to ride it out. Afterward, the survivors emerge to assess the damage, if there is any. No matter what your circumstances are, you are a survivor of whatever life has dealt you. You have survived the tornado of your past and it is time to come from the basement and assess the damage, if there is any.

To assess the truth about how life is going for you *right now*, we will look at your current level of health, happiness, and prosperity (HHP). We do this by examining various aspects of the four essential requirements of a constructive life (awareness, wellness, relationships, and resources) to determine what level of fulfillment you have in each area. This will give you a summary analysis of your reality, including any good, bad, hidden, or obvious information.

Although each person's desired HHP level is different, most humans require at least the baseline comfort of a healthy and protected body. That baseline usually includes access to healthy food and clean water; sufficient physical use of the body; manageable stress levels; protection from environmental factors like excessive heat, cold, dryness, and humidity; protection from destructive forces like toxicities and hurricanes; and access to the knowledge, tools, and resources needed to maintain and/or move beyond these baselines.

Some people require nothing more than these basic needs to reach their desired HHP levels, and life is fine for them. Others, however, have the need to continuously evolve and improve in the four key areas.

Step 2 of your journey to HealthyIsm asks you to take a thorough and honest look at all aspects of your life, in which interconnected, synergistic parts participate in co-creating and co-maintaining the condition of your body and mind. You will do this by using a series of affirmations to *analyze your reality,* taking care to be as honest as you possibly can.

The affirmations in this step are divided into four categories:

1. Calm Awareness: How aware are you of the way you think and act and of what's happening around you and in the world? Do you make choices and take actions consciously or unconsciously?

2. Well Body, Mind, and Soul: Do you give yourself the right elements to develop and maintain your physical, mental, and spiritual bodies?

3. Nurtured Relationships: What is your relationship level with self, significant other, family, other people, charities, plants and animals, and spirituality?

4. Building and Maintaining Resources: What tools, resources, and assets do you have to work with, such as good health, business sense, knowledge, talents, physical strength, languages, and global connectivity?

The following analysis of your life is done using affirmations, because when you affirm something you logically and/or intuitively know if that statement is true, partially true, or not at all. Using the chart at the end of this chapter to record your findings, identify how you rank on a scale of 1 (strongly disagree) to 10 (strongly agree) for each affirmation below. (Take affirmation #3 under Calm Awareness, for example: if I strongly disagreed with the statement "I am calmly aware of my IMP..." I'd give myself a ranking of 1. If I strongly agreed, I'd give myself a 10. If I was vaguely aware that I behaved a certain way because of parental or religious programming, I'd give myself a ranking in between.) As you read each affirmation, mark your ranking in the column next to the number. When you have finished, transfer the rankings to the Step 2 exercise sheet at the end of the chapter.

Remember that the affirmations listed here are based on the author's own life and intended goals; therefore, use them as a guide, eliminating some and adding others wherever you feel it's necessary. The goal is to look at your own life, be honest with what you see, record your findings, and give yourself a report. After you have finished the book and applied all the recommended steps, come back and reanalyze your HHP level. Odds are that there will be some—possibly spectacular—improvements in your life.

(Note: See Chapter 10 for further explanation of each affirmation.)

Let's get started! Read the following affirmations and mark your score.

Calm Awareness

1. Without having to actually "think" about it, I am calmly aware of this exact moment and of everything going on inside and around me. I'm aware of my lungs, heart, and body. I'm aware of my visual surroundings, the sounds near and far, the smells, and the "energy" emitted by other people. I'm calmly aware of the presence of plants and animals, the earth below, and the universe above.

2. I am calmly aware of the obvious and hidden agendas and beliefs of others like advertisers, government, various media, religious institutions, and the educational system.

3. I am calmly aware of my programmed mind, my IMP, how it controls my life, and how it has generally developed my personal core values.

4. I am calmly aware that what I ingest affects my mind biologically and, therefore, my thinking. Healthy foods equal clarity; garbage foods equal mental fogginess.

5. I am calmly aware that what I ingest affects my physical energy and physical results, such as a healthy body or a body laden with health problems.

6. I am calmly aware of my body's physical messages. When something aches or I have an illness, I endeavor to discover the root of the problem so I can treat the cause and not the symptom.

7. I am calmly aware of the meal in front of me, acknowledging and appreciating its life force in the nutrients it gives to me.

8. I am calmly aware of my connectivity to a higher source, be it God or a Universal Spirit.

9. I am calmly aware of my "general purpose" as a human, which is to participate in the evolutionary process itself.

10. I am calmly aware of my "specific purpose" as a human.

11. I have identified and am calmly aware of my direction in life.

12. I am calmly aware of death as a natural part of a universal biological process and thus do not fear death but do welcome living healthily to an old age. I recognize that deep sadness for a lost loved one is a natural primal reaction but that I must not allow it to take away from my quality of life and the welcoming in of great health, happiness, and prosperity.

13. I am calmly aware of survival instincts that affect my life and how, if they are not controlled, they may be destructive to self or others. (See Chapter 5 to review information on destructive instincts).

14. I am calmly aware that my body operates on different rhythms, including day and night, seasonal, and hormonal.

15. I am calmly aware of silver linings—that good things can often be found in bad circumstances.

16. I am calmly aware that there is a global shift in consciousness toward a collectively constructive HHP world rather than a continuance of the many destructive aspects of the present.

F.E.A.R.:
Focus on an **E**xperience/Expectation **A**ffecting **R**eality

We all know people who always seem to be afraid of or worried about just about everything. Fear reduces one's quality of life either by draining energy from constructive thinking and action or by causing unnecessary stress in the moment because of potential negative outcomes.

Fear is a **F**ocus on a potential problem or danger of a current **E**xperience (or future Expectation) **A**ffecting **R**eality.

For example, for a person with a fear of flying, the evidence is true, not false, that a plane can cause injury or death. The focus on that expected threat negatively affects the person's present moment and creates real emotions. So the feeling he gets is not caused by false evidence or emotions; it's more about a pessimistic focus on things that might happen.

Because of our instincts and inner mental programming, many of our lives are dictated by fear. A person may have a great idea but focuses on reasons why it wouldn't work, feels the emotion caused by that focus, and stops the idea in its tracks. Or life may be beautiful, but that person focuses on the expectation that something terrible might happen.

Do any of these statements of F.E.A.R. sound familiar?
- "I will not get close to this new person because I'm afraid this relationship will end up like the last one."
- "I will not bother to get healthy because I don't want to look strange in front of my friends."
- "I will not try to put my idea into action because I'm afraid it's not good enough."
- "I will not let my child go to play with a friend because something terrible could happen when I'm not there."

Fear is most likely a combination of a survival instinct (like the constant vigilance of a deer in the woods) and nurtured programming (like the constant fear Mom has about spiders or what might happen next Tuesday).

If you are going to focus on things that **might** happen, have a positive outlook; have faith and trust that you will attain great HHP. That doesn't mean ignore possible dangers but rather face threats with calm awareness and constructive thinking. It's less stressful and much healthier!

Well Body, Mind, and Soul

1. I know that my body is designed for many physical functions like pushing, pulling, walking, and running, and I know how much and which types of exercise are right for *my* body.

2. I give all the muscles in my body just enough use, movement, and/or exercise.

3. I give my body and mind the proper fuel to get and stay healthy. I know which foods/fuel are "right" for *my* body and understand the nutrient density of the foods I eat. I also give my body enough daily intake of water.

4. I give my body just enough of the "right" foods/fuel.

5. I give my body just enough sunshine on a daily basis, if available.

6. I keep my body "clean," meaning that it is free from the toxins in my food and in my environment.

7. I am in control of my treats and indulgences, including my intake of unhealthy foods, drugs, and alcohol.

8. I challenge my mind regularly with activities like crossword puzzles, riddles, and problem solving.

9. I feed my mind with "good" information about the best foods, the best exercises for my body, the best way to invest my money, and so on.

10. I meditate/pray often and find moments to be with myself and/or God/Universal Spirit.

11. I get enough sleep every night; I try to go to bed soon after the sun goes down and get up soon after it rises.

12. I have quiet time daily to rest my mind and body. My quiet time may or may not be in conjunction with my times of meditation/prayer.

13. I find time to laugh, dance, sing, and play on a regular basis, preferably daily.

14. I am in tune with my emotions, where they are coming from, and what messages they are delivering to me.

Nurtured Relationships

1. I have a great relationship with the most important person—myself. That means I forgive myself for my "mess-ups" and accept and love myself at whatever level I am at.

2. My relationship with my significant other is loving, trusting, tolerant, and patient. We enjoy a comfortable level of compatibility yet have enough diversity to keep our relationship spicy. If our relationship needs to be improved upon, I first look within myself.

3. My relationship with my coworkers, employees, and/or boss is congenial and mutually beneficial. It is pleasant to work with them, and I look forward to seeing them every day.

4. My relationships with my immediate family, children, parents, and/or siblings are full of mutual love, patience, and tolerance, and I communicate effectively with all of them.

5. I have a kind, respectful, and loving relationship with the earth and its creatures and plants, and I have a low or nonexistent ecological footprint.

6. My relationship with God/Universal Spirit is strong, loving, forgiving, and rewarding.

7. I have good relationships with my neighbors, my community, and all the people of this great earth. I look others in the eye and am helpful to them. Regardless of background or beliefs, I feel like I am part of a large brotherhood.

8. I am charitable toward others and generous with money, time, resources, and physical energies. I strive to create relationships with those in real need of my support.

Building and Maintaining Resources

1. I am in control of my biggest resource of all—my

thoughts. My thoughts always start from a place of gratitude for all the good things in my life, and I use them to create a constructive reality.

2. I ask myself focused, positive, good questions that, in finding the answers, improve my life or the lives of others.

3. I have good communications skills. I am able to communicate what I want to others and to understand what others communicate to me.

4. I enjoy good health, which helps me in every other area of my life.

5. I recognize and am in tune with my intuition and "gut feelings" and have acted upon those feelings in the past.

6. I have a support network of family, friends, and community that I can rely on when in need.

7. I am wise and have general and/or specific experience in certain areas that helps me make decisions as I move through life.

8. I have innate talents, strengths, and/or skills, and I use them.

9. I have a job or profession that I like and that provides me with satisfactory payment.

10. I am professionally and personally productive and pro-

duce things that are good for me and the earth or that at least have a neutral effect.

11. I have assets in the form of cashable items or land.

12. I have a place where I can regularly "get away from it all."

13. I have tools like a car, computer, and other equipment that help me in other areas of my life.

14. I have willpower, and if I set my mind to something, I usually complete it.

15. I have it locked into my brain that all transgressions against me, even those I do against myself, are ultimately to be forgiven.

16. I continually get rid of clutter in my head, my closet, my house, and my life, which eliminates barriers to positive change and growth.

17. I use the Internet to be globally connected, to receive or offer messages and knowledge, and/or to receive or offer products and services.

18. I have a healthy amount of stress in my life that keeps me on my toes physically, emotionally, and mentally so that I do not become weak, flabby, unchallenged, or dull.

19. I have a means, such as exercise or meditation, of "healthily" releasing or controlling the stress in my life.

20. I am a truthful person who always comes from a place of truth.

21. I am able to defend myself, or at least have the chance to do so, when attacked or cornered. I also defend myself by choosing with calm awareness to walk on safer streets both physically and metaphorically.

22. When and if I choose to do so, I allow the sacrifice of various aspects of my own health, happiness, and prosperity in order to help others who are committed to positively evolving.

23. I use time as a tool to construct a healthy life rather than as a weapon to destroy myself with unhealthy habits.

24. I use the earth in a healthy and beneficial way by sustaining its resources even as I gratefully and lovingly use them for air, food, water, energy, and land.

25. I am peaceful with self and others as often as possible.

26. I move outside of my safety zone and take occasional calculated risks.

27. I make conscious choices about who I vote for and where I spend my money as a way to influence corporate and government HealthyIsm.

28. I am clear as to what I want to welcome into my life.

Yes, a lot to think about and perhaps a bit mentally tiring. If it is tiring, that's okay; it's part of the process. Don't overdo it; proceed at your own pace. Just as you must go through various stages in any project (gather information, develop a plan, gather resources, and take action) you must do the same with project "Healthy I." You are in the beginning stage of gathering information. In analyzing the four distinct requirements of a constructive life you now have lots of data about your current truth. With this reality check of what's happening in your life right now, good or bad, it's time for the next step, which is still gathering information, but this time you'll review your history to see what has contributed to the life you live today, good or bad.

Step 2 Exercise: Determine Your HHP Level

Record the rankings you wrote next to each affirmation in Step 2. (Copy this page first so you can do another ranking at a later time.)

Date: _____

Calm Awareness			
1.	5.	9.	13.
2.	6.	10.	14.
3.	7.	11.	15.
4.	8.	12	16.
Total Calm Awareness Ranking _____			

Well Body, Mind, and Soul			
1.	5.	9.	13.
2.	6.	10.	14.
3.	7.	11.	
4.	8.	12	
Total Wellness Ranking _____			

Nurtured Relationships			
1.	3.	5.	7.
2.	4.	6.	8.
Total Relationships Ranking _____			

Building and Maintaining Resources			
1.	8.	15.	22.
2.	9.	16.	23.
3.	10.	17.	24.
4.	11.	18.	25.
5.	12.	19.	26.
6.	13.	20.	27.
7.	14.	21.	28.
Total Resources Ranking _____			

    Current HHP Level _____
    (Add the totals from each category)

You have now completed Step 2. Mark this chapter and this page, as you will come back to it in Step 6.

Step 3: Zoom Out — Review Your Overall Past

"You have to know the past to understand the present."
—Dr. Carl Sagan

"If we could read the secret history of our enemies, we should find in each man's life sorrow and suffering enough to disarm all hostility."
—Henry Wadsworth Longfellow

"Those who cannot remember the past are condemned to repeat it."
—George Santayana

Now that you have had a look at the underlying causes of your Unhealthyolic lifestyle—like our destructive instincts and IMP, which control the way we think—and you have truthfully looked at what's going on in your life *now*, it's time to zoom out to review and focus on what you know or remember about your *past*.

In Step 1 we took a global view of what happened to humanity as a whole and looked at the inner mental programming and various instincts that cause us to act and think the way we do. In Step 2 you emerged from the basement to examine the truth about your own present-day reality.

In Step 3, you will do the important work of focusing more on the past *I* to understand the experiences, influences, and interactions, good or bad, that made you who you are today. You will try to connect past experiences and guidance (whether it was parental, schooling, societal, or any of the other reasons described in Step 1) that contribute to your current good habits of living a healthy, happy, and prosperous life or that are responsible for most of your Unhealthyolic habits.

You will use this personal history in the next chapter, Step 4, where you'll focus strictly on the destructive components, the messy past issues, of your list. Then, in Step 5, you'll use a method that will help you *fix* whatever has led you down an unhealthy path and offer yourself some *relief*.

Remember to also include good or bad things that you have done *for* or *to* others. For example, if you helped an old lady cross the street and you remember her smiling with teary eyes, record that. Conversely, if you hurt someone physically or verbally, even if in *justified* retaliation, record that.

Remember When

As you work through this exercise and visit the historic you, remember that even one second ago is the old you—so any memory at all is fair game! Your goal is to review and record your life in order to identify the things that influenced how you think and act.

To start, use the blank page at the end of this chapter or bring up a blank document on your computer so you can create a numbered list of memories. Begin with the most recent event in your life (#1) and work your way back to your earliest memory (#?). Keep your focus and attention directed on what you remember, even if it's vague, and be sure to include both good and bad memories.

Here are some ideas to jog your memory and help get you started:

- Memories at different periods in your life: as a toddler, a young child, a pre-teen, a teenager, a young adult, and so on

- A good or bad experience with a spouse, child, extended family member, or other person (a relaxing vacation, an argument)

- Parents telling you to do or not do something

- Specific lessons learned from teachers, religious leaders, professors, or business mentors

- An important event

- An experience you had with (or knowledge you have about) your culture, such as "we always have a weekly cultural dinner together" or "my culture disowned me because of my pregnancy out of wedlock"

- What someone said or did to you and your reaction to it

- What you did to someone and his/her reaction to it

- Thoughts you had about another person's actions or ideas

- A pleasant or unpleasant, conscious or unconscious, emotion or feeling you had (happy, sad, surprised, mad, disgusted, fearful) and what caused it.

Don't get bogged down in details, complete sentences, or good grammar—just jot down a word or phrase that represents the memory or knowledge. For example, if one of your earliest memories is running through a field laughing with your mother, you can just write "running and laughing in field with Mom."

Case Study

Here's a case study to further illustrate how to record your personal history. Our subject is Sally, a 40-year-old, depressed, obese mother of two obese teenagers who are also depressed. During the exercise, Sally remembers many key experiences and influences in her life, as well as seemingly inconsequential moments that have nonetheless made an impression on her.

Following is a sampling of Sally's memories:

#1. stranger smiled at me *(Sally's most recent memory was of a moment yesterday when a stranger held open a door for her at the bank and smiled sincerely.)*

> **Remember...**
>
> *When recording your life, start with the most recent events and work backward as far as you can.*

#2. husband yelled, called me fat *(Here Sally describes an event last month when she and her husband argued about the bad health and depression of their children.)*

#22. cranky children, food to calm *(Sally remembers feeling overwhelmed by her two cranky, fussy toddlers, and how she placated them with food. She remembers eating to calm herself down as well.)*

#31. Father O'Callahan warning me *(Sally remembers the priest telling her, when she was a teenager, that she would not go to heaven if she didn't listen to her parents.)*

#42. Mom made me eat my supper *(Here Sally remembers that her mother, who was raised the same way, always forced Sally and her siblings to eat everything on their plates.)*

#43. field, laughing, Mom *(Sally records her wonderful*

memories of playing and running in a field somewhere, with her mother playfully chasing after her.)

#47. told dad that I hated him *(Sally remembers the hurt look on her father's face when her 10-year-old self told him that she hated him and wished he was dead.)*

#51. father yelling, hitting mother *(Sally remembers a time when she was six that she and her little sister were awakened by yelling. Gathered at the top of the stairs, they saw their dad yelling at and hitting their mother.)*

#58. father playing with me in a playground (Sally remembers one of the few times her father played with her when she was a toddler.)

This exercise may be an emotional roller coaster for you as you relive your past (if you are suffering mentally please consult a professional.) We will work on relieving ourselves of mental baggage in Steps 4 and 5. What is most important to remember right now is *to love and accept yourself as you are.* Some of your past may have created your destructive IMP and set you on an Unhealthyolic path, but you're now ready to take control and get constructive!

Step 3 Exercise: Review Your History

As you reviewed your history, did you notice particular experiences and influences, either good or bad, which affect the way you are today? Use this page to record your most profound discoveries.

Step 4: Zoom In – Reveal Your Messy Past

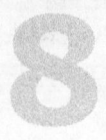

Who controls the past controls the future: who controls the present controls the past.
—George Orwell

Every saint has a past and every sinner has a future.
—Oscar Wilde

Only by acceptance of the past, can you alter it.
—T. S. Eliot

Now that you've got a list of your good and bad memories and knowledge in front of you, you must face the things that just were not constructive to your life. After all, before we can fix something, we have to recognize that it's broken. Step 4 is an important exercise in which you will identify and focus on the "broken parts" by zooming in on the negative guidance, experiences, and memories that may be influencing your Unhealthyolic habits today and preventing your future of HHP.

What Issues?

Do you have any experiences from your past that are affecting you mentally today? It's time to reflect and recognize any past issues that negatively controls you today. Go down your list that you worked on in the last chapter with a highlighter or pencil in hand and mark all the problems, broken parts, and messy areas. You may have already flagged a few that were emotional or obviously destructive. As you go through the list you may remember other negative experiences; write those down also. This will become your personal fix-it list—those things that need your attention as you continue on the road to HealthyIsm. In Chapter 5 we will work on freeing yourself from any control these memories have over your life today.

As you develop your messy memory list, be sure to look for and include the following:

What others have done to you

- Bullies of any kind who inflicted physical, verbal, or mental abuse on you at any point in your life, from youth to adulthood. The abuse could be from an individual or an institution. For example, suppose you refused to vaccinate your kids because doing so went against your moral judgment. If you didn't know you had a legal right not to vaccinate based on your religious or moral beliefs, you might have suffered verbal and mental abuse in the form of threats from your local government.

- "Good intention abuse," such as parents forcing you to eat when you weren't hungry, thereby making your eating experience stressful rather than peaceful and spiritual. Or a well-meaning institution that passed on to you their destructive beliefs.

- Any tragic event, such as being hit by a drunk driver, that caused physical damage or worse to you or your family.

What you have done to others

- Have you inflicted physical, verbal, or mental abuse on others? We are not born with the intent to harm others, but as we grow, so does our IMP—and its control of our minds may cause us to do nasty things. Our primal urges also make us do nasty things like "snarling" at others when they threaten to take our objects of survival like food, water, shelter, or mates.

- Have you ever stolen from others?

- Have you ever said terrible things to others? Do you remember their reaction?

- Have you ever hurt someone out of anger or frustration?

- Have you inflicted good intention abuse? This comes in many shapes, such as forcing your children to eat or mowing a neighbor's lawn only to discover that you inadvertently mowed down some precious plants he'd been nurturing. Or has your company that you built from the ground up harmed others or the earth in its sincere quest to maximize profits and provide employment for many people?

What you have done to yourself

- Have you hurt yourself physically, verbally, or mentally? Have you ever done things to yourself consciously or unconsciously that have turned out to be harmful? For example, you might have followed the general nutrition guideline of the past that advocated a low-fat diet with plenty of "low-fat" breads and pastas. Then later you discovered that your body needed more of that fat and less of those grains—and that "healthy" diet may be the cause of the aches, pains, and diseases you have now.

- After doing something stupid, have you ever called yourself names or punished yourself with grief, guilt, or shame?

- As a teenager, did you drink alcohol and do drugs recreationally and then find yourself in the future relying on a daily fix in order to function?

Problems with personal, social, and work relationships

- Has your life been negatively affected by certain actions or teachings of your parents, such as being fiercely scolded for spilling milk or being told something like "money is evil?"

- Do you fear your neighbors or the people of your city because of the chaos you see daily on the news shows—when in reality, 99.9% of your neighbors are good, well-intentioned people?

- Do you mistrust all of your coworkers because you were once harmed by a coworker who made a flawed decision?

Dogmas and beliefs that have slowed your growth

- Did any dogma, belief, or teaching from other people, a particular culture, or institutions cause you to act destructively or instill you with fear, shame, guilt, or anger?

Start Your Personal Fix-It List

The goal of this "cleaning house" exercise is to identify those things that are out of balance in your life and that are not supporting your optimal evolution. Creating this list should also help you recognize the past guidance, experiences, and memories that are messy enough to control you today. When you know what's broken you can successfully confront and remedy the situation. The hope is that these problem areas are immediately revealed to you, not in a "change or else" way, but in a kind and nurturing way that will ease you down the road to healthy, constructive habits.

Now that you've identified the problems or "messy" areas, you'll need to devise a plan to fix them and put your personal world into some helpful order. In the next chapter, we will explore a method of releasing the control these past messy areas have over you, leaving ample room to evolve and build a helpful, constructive life.

Step 4 Exercise: Personal Fix-It List

From your highlighted memories, choose the messy memories you would like to fix and write them in below. Use extra sheets of paper as necessary.

1. MESSY MEMORY:

2. MESSY MEMORY:

3. MESSY MEMORY:

4. MESSY MEMORY:

5. MESSY MEMORY:

6. MESSY MEMORY:

7. MESSY MEMORY:

8. MESSY MEMORY:

9. MESSY MEMORY:

HealthyIsm: *Healthy I, Healthy World!*

10. MESSY MEMORY:

11. MESSY MEMORY:

12. MESSY MEMORY:

13. MESSY MEMORY:

14. MESSY MEMORY:

Step 5: R.E.L.I.E.F.!

There are two sighs of relief every night in the life of an opera manager. The first comes when the curtain goes up. The second sigh of relief comes when the final curtain goes down without any disaster, and one realizes, gratefully, that the miracle has happened again.
– Rudolf Bing

And thou wilt give thyself relief, if thou doest every act of thy life as if it were the last.
– Marcus Aurelius

For fast acting relief, try slowing down.
– Lily Tomlin

So far on your journey to overcoming destructive habits and then welcoming a life of HealthyIsm, you've been asked to consider a few major questions:

- Does your IMP cause any problems in your life?

- Do any particular evolutionary instincts also contribute to those problems?

- Are there any messy memories that still influence your present reality?

Now it's time for Step 5: R.E.L.I.E.F. (**R**ecord **E**vent, **L**et go, **I**nsert **E**verlasting **F**orgiveness), in which you welcome relief by recognizing and releasing the manipulators that control your life. The "event" could be any messy memory, experience, IMP, or instinct. This process includes letting go of these events and forgiving yourself and others for any contribution to your destructive state. The ultimate goal is to direct all your energies toward a life of thinking and acting constructively.

> **Constructive Creation...**
>
> *You can't change yesterday. You can only acknowledge it, learn from it, and forgive it if necessary. You can, however, change your tomorrow by being aware of the manipulators that dictate your thinking and actions, take control, and constructively create your TODAY.*

Think again about how most babies are before they are programmed. If their diapers are clean and they are fed and loved, then they are peaceful, loving, happy, and always living in the moment—until we distract them, that is, as we were programmed to do. When a baby is eating, playing with pots, constructing language, or mimicking your facial expressions, he is always in the moment. We are naturally attracted to these bundles of joy, as if they represent a glimpse of a primal part of ourselves that wants to be freely in the moment. It's time to relieve ourselves of the things that use to, and still do, distract us from constructing a comfortable world.

Building Blocks

The work of relieving yourself of your Unhealthyolic habits and restoring every realm of your life to HealthyIsm is created with the building blocks of awareness, forgiveness, self-acceptance, and unconditional love. Before beginning this work, let's consider a few questions:

- **Do you need to become aware to restore your life?** Yes! If you continue blindly on the same path, you'll keep arriving at the same place. There is an obvious mess in the world and perhaps in your own life, too. You need to be aware of the path that brought you there and then find or develop another path. Your awareness starts with knowing your destructive instincts and the control your IMP has over your life.

- **Do you need others to forgive you?** That would be nice because you may sense some good energy, but the answer is no! The desire for forgiveness from others is based on low self-esteem, shame, or guilt. Remember that you cannot control the actions, thoughts, and reactions of others, so it's best to rise above that need for forgiveness and reverse it. If you did do something that hurt or upset another person, say you're sorry and mean it!

- **Do you need to forgive others?** Yes! There is a wonderful saying that not forgiving others is like drinking poison and expecting the other person to die. Most religions encourage forgiveness in one way or another. Even so, it's not necessary to forget immediately, or at all, unless you feel weak and experience negative feelings that rise to the surface when you remember a past event; in that case, it's best to forget or put the emotion away to deal with when you are stronger. But, for your health and the health of humanity, you must at least forgive! In any forgive/forget situation, ask yourself what you learned, what you could have done differently, and what you will do differently in the future if a similar situation arises—then move on!

- **Do you need to forgive yourself?** Yes! Instead of regretting past thoughts, actions, or inactions, or beating yourself up because you fell into the trap of destructive instincts or IMP, you must forgive yourself completely and unconditionally. And again, ask yourself what you have learned. Gandhi's quote "hate the sin, love the sinner" can be applied equally to others and to yourself—you don't have to forgive the act or the thought or the habit that consumes you, but you do have to forgive every part of your being.

- **Do you need to be open to receive love or give love to recover?** Yes! When someone sends you love, receive it with open arms as you would receive the sun on the first warm, spring day. And to give love unconditionally means that we are in love with ourselves. Receiving and giving love pulls us towards the higher states of consciousness of joy and peace. With love will come a healthy I and a healthy world.[23]

- **Do you need to accept yourself the way you are?** Yes! That's your starting point. Your destructive thinking may need repairing, but you are perfect as you are. Wherever you are in your physical, mental, and spiritual growth may not be perfect in the eyes of other humans, but that's their own IMP talking. Your current position in life is the starting point where you can welcome a life of HealthyIsm. As Shayne (my pseudo-adopted, cheerful, successful son who lost both his legs, one hand, and the tops of all his fingers on the remaining hand) would put it: "I'm just differently capable." No two people are alike; wherever you are in life, you are "differently *capable*" and perfect!

- **Do you need help from others?** It certainly doesn't hurt! Welcoming a life of HealthyIsm is like trying to build a house by yourself—you can do it, but the work goes faster and is much more enjoyable when you've got someone by your side.

- **Do you need help from Universal Spirit or God?** Once you decide to help yourself through a program like the one described in this book, Universal Spirit/God will kick in its fair share automatically—almost miraculously! However, being an aware person, you know that it's not a miracle at all: it's just the natural law of the universe that when we are open to receive and we have our focus on something that "feels" right, and we take constructive action, it has a better chance of "coming to us." Some call it the law of attraction; HealthyIsm calls it the "law of constructive thinking and action."

- **Do you need to "fix" everything at once?** No. Go at your own pace. You can work on all the negative stuff in your life and succeed, but you can also start small with one habit or one unhealthy, implanted belief at a time. What will happen is that each time you move on to the next belief or habit, you'll be a bit stronger than the last time and the habit will be easier to deal with. It'll be as if you've been given a homeopathic dose or vaccine for overcoming habits that strengthens your "habit-breaking" system.

So, just how do you live this life of forgiveness, acceptance, and love? How do you build a life of great HHP? In considering the information in the previous chapters and having done Steps 1 through 4, you have done most of the work already! Now it's time for the R.E.L.I.E.F. technique to get rid of all that heavy mental baggage you've been carrying around with you.

The R.E.L.I.E.F. Technique

R.E.L.I.E.F. (**R**ecord **E**vent, **L**et go, **I**nsert **E**verlasting **F**orgiveness) is a technique for stopping the negative controllers of your life so that you can welcome great HHP. (Remember that an event can also be any messy memory, experience, IMP, or instinct).

The goal is to minimize or completely let go of any hold that negative events may have over you. It is about releasing any destructive levels of consciousness, such as fear, low self-esteem, guilt, shame, anger, etc., so that you can concentrate your energies on welcoming love, happiness, peace, prosperity, and good health. In short, the goal is to be conscious of any manipulative thinking patterns so that you can take control and practice living more constructively.

Before going through the following exercise, familiarize yourself with the sample R.E.L.I.E.F. list table at the end of this chapter.

Then go to the blank list table and fill it in as you go through the steps. Make copies of the blank table first so that you have plenty of room to add all the messy stuff from your past and in your life now. Okay, here we go:

Step 5 Exercise: R.E.L.I.E.F. Instructions
(Use With Blank Table At End Of Chapter):

Record Event

1. Referring to the Personal Fix-It List you created in Step 4, record each messy memory in the first column on the blank R.E.L.I.E.F. list.

2. In addition to this list of messy memories, record any

other destructive events, experiences, IMP, or instincts, that you are aware of, each in its own box. As you record, label each box as a messy memory, event, IMP, etc., or a combination such as a mixture of IMP and instinct.

3. In the second column, under Resultant Emotion, record any emotion that you may feel now or remember feeling. Since we are working on "messy stuff" most emotions will be negative; but occasionally you may have a seemingly positive emotion, such as feeling happy because you received praise for emulating your father's perception of the world.

4. In the third column, Adds to Which Destructive Habit, if it becomes clear to you that a current destructive habit is the result of the destructive events in the first column, record it. For example, if you automatically act aggressively toward people "not like you" because your sister taught you to ridicule or assault other cultures and different skin colors, record it in the third column.

5. In the last column, Reasons I Continue Destructive Habit; Notes, record any possible reasons or illusory benefits that contribute to you continuing your destructive habits. If you smoke or eat junk food to soothe your mind, for example, you might write "this destructive habit relaxes me," or "it conjures up good feelings and good memories." You could also place a note here for any other thought that comes to mind, such as "I must practice my religion on my own terms."

6. Take your time and go wild! Make the exercise a "re-

CHAPTER 9. STEP 5: R.E.L.I.E.F.!

play-storming session." As with a brainstorming session, allow *all* the stuff that comes up to be recorded without worrying whether or not it should be on the list.

> **Ya Gotta Forgive!**
>
> *Forgiveness plays a large part in succeeding in your quest for HealthyIsm. Not forgiving will just make you sick in many ways. To move forward, you must forgive all past transgressions done unto you by others, done unto others by you, and—most importantly—done unto you by YOU!*

7. Don't worry about being perfect. If you forget things or write down things that "shouldn't" be there, that's okay! Just becoming aware of the destructive memories, events, experiences, IMP, or instincts is enough to allow *all* destructive aspects of your life (past or present) to control you no more. But for ease of mind, record as the last entry in your list a blanket statement, such as "Any *other* destructive memory, event, experience, IMP, or instinct". See bottom of sample R.E.L.I.E.F. list at the end of the chapter.

Let go

8. Time to let go of the control that these destructive manipulators have over your life. When you think you are done with your list, stop, free up your hands, and relax (if you're not sure if you're done, it's okay; you can always add to your list later and do the exercise again, if you recall additional stuff).

9. Welcome getting out of your head for a minute, ceasing all thoughts, connecting with your body, and becoming grounded. Sitting tall and comfortably (or lying down, if you prefer), place your hands in a comfortable position and take a few deep breaths. Without using your hands, feel your heartbeat and pulse. When you find it, imagine your pulse as the pulsation of something larger than you but also within you, the pulse of God or Universal Spirit or of Consciousness itself. (If you don't like nor need the spiritual stuff, that's okay. Just continue with the rest of the exercise.) Now imagine that you have roots of energy emerging downward from your body and rooting into the earth below. Envision a cocoon of peaceful, beautiful energy surrounding your body and connecting upward with the cosmos above. With this clear vision of roots below, connection above, and your breath and pulse representing something larger, feel your mind and body merging with all that is. If your mind wanders, that's okay; just bring your mind back into your next breath and pulse. Continue practicing this state for a couple of minutes or more.

10. From this grounded state, pick up the list you just made, read through it, and observe your thoughts and feelings. Observe your destructive IMP desperately trying to keep control of your life. Gently say things like, "Hello, IMP. The game is over. I will not need you anymore. I am aware now. I have outgrown your control over my life. I am in control now."

11. Recognize the control that all the "stuff" on your list has had *and still* has on your current thinking and actions, and then *welcome letting go.* That's right—let go of the

control that these manipulators have! NOW! Talk to your constructive self. Tell it that no event, experience, emotion, IMP, instinct, messy memory, or anything else will drain energy from your life any more. You have better uses for all your energies! You are reserving them for constructive thinking and action. Say thank you to the past stuff for making you stronger or for providing you with silver linings. Now say goodbye. You might even say it with a slight smile, as if you were bidding farewell to old acquaintances who only brought you trouble. (If you find some areas that you just can't let go of, that's okay. Put them aside for further work with a professional therapist, and move on to the next step if you can.)

Insert Everlasting Forgiveness

12. Now that your unwelcome mental guests have left, it's time to insert everlasting forgiveness into your thinking. As you continue with this exercise, acknowledge that, first and foremost, you are forgiving for you. When you forgive, you are removing any further burdens and acquiring even more energy toward a constructive life. Insert everlasting forgiveness into your thoughts about *everyone and everything* that ever caused destruction in your life. Forgive all the stuff on your list and any institutions or people that were involved. If you think of someone or something else to forgive, record it anywhere on the page. Remember to forgive yourself for any involvement. Now mark in large letters across your entire list "I FORGIVE!" Pause for a moment and feel the weight lifting off of you.

13. From this place of awareness, of everlasting forgiveness, of freedom, take your list of manipulators and *rip it up.* Tear the list into tiny bits and put it in a dustpan or container for transportation to its final destination. Take these corpses of the old manipulators in your life and bury them directly in the ground next to any plant to be absorbed and assimilated by nature just as manure feeds a plant. Make it a ceremony that is sweeter than sorrow.

Wash and Rinse

14. Once you've finished your burial, it's time to symbolically *wash and rinse* any lingering residue of destructive manipulators. First, pretend that you are washing your whole body, lathering every part of the body with a special soap that will clean away any remaining residue. Once you have completed a head-to-toe wash, go over your whole body again; this time, however, *rinse* using a sweeping action of your hand to brush away any residue. Even though this exercise may seem strange, it is very important to perform. You are subconsciously cleaning your mind of anything that drains you of energy, which you will need to constructively welcome into your life great HHP.

15. Now that you are *clean,* look into a mirror from only a few inches away and focus just on your eyes. Recognize and welcome your primal self deep inside, the part that flourishes when it lives *in* the moment. Repeat affirmations aloud to yourself, through your eyes, such as:

    • "Congratulations for letting go."

CHAPTER 9. STEP 5: R.E.L.I.E.F.!

- "You are now clean...free."

- "I accept and love you as you are."

- "You are a good person."

- "I forgive you."

- "I feel great without those mental manipulators!"

- "I am in control of my destructive thoughts... forever!"

- "I welcome a constructive life."

16. When you are done with the mirror and affirmations, pause, take a deep breath, and relax. Welcome your mental *freedom,* take a break, and then move on!

> **Remember...**
>
> *The goal of this R.E.L.I.E.F. work is to identify and control your instincts and IMP, learn to stop Unhealthyolic habits, welcome HHP, and think thoughts that support your evolution and the evolution of others and the planet.*

How you make (and destroy) this list is really up to you. Design your own ceremony. Perhaps you'd prefer to record your list on a computer, and then hit the delete button. If you're artistic, maybe you'd rather draw, paint, or sculpt a non-verbal "list"—and then destroy it. The important thing is just to do it.

(If you do come up with a different method that works for you, we'd love to know about it! Log into the forums on the HealthyIsm.com website and join the "R.E.L.I.E.F." thread.)

You do not have to destroy the list; you can keep a copy for future reference if you like. The goal of this exercise is not to ignore what happened in the past, but rather to free yourself from the mental control it has in your life today and going forward—and to further empower *you* to stop your Unhealthyolic habits.

When you become aware and relieve yourself of any destructive events that influence your present thinking, you will once again be able to live freely *in* the moment. It will not only feel great, you will be setting an example for many others to do the same: healthy *I*, healthy world.

Once you evolve to being aware of those things that affect your life, you will *forever be aware* and in better control of your life. What was hidden or unconscious to you before will now always be apparent. With practice, no event, and no person marketing their perception of reality, will be able to control your HHP.

This whole HealthyIsm process may at first seem strange and intolerable. Eventually, however—and sooner than you think—your new habits and lifestyle will become not just tolerable, but a matter of routine and enjoyable.

Living unconsciously can create destructive habits that foster fear, jealousy, victimization, judgment, and emptiness. To move beyond all that, you need to become aware of that destructiveness and then adopt an attitude that is on the other side of the same coin: constructive habits that bring calm, trust, responsibility, acceptance, and abundance. When you do that, you eliminate undesirable attitudes at the same time that you adopt desirable ones, because they cannot coexist.

When you are working for the greater good of all mankind, you cannot possibly be simultaneously working *against* it. Lucky for us, the two mindsets represent a dichotomy, two contradictory ideas that you cannot get inside your head or inside your life at the same time.

This chapter presents just one alternative method of relieving the past's hold on your present and future. The R.E.L.I.E.F. technique used here is incredibly effective, but some people may find further help in such other unconventional forms as acupuncture, NLP (neuro-linguistic programming) techniques, EFT (emotional freedom techniques), or working conventionally with an open-minded medical professional. The whole intent is to move forward into a life of constructive consciousness with as little (or no) baggage as possible to hold you back. (For more information on other techniques, visit www.HealthyIsm.com.)

Throughout this process, you may experience inevitable slips, regressions, and setbacks. Although that may not be the case for everyone, if you do have a setback, remember to still exercise self-compassion and forgiveness. When you do experience a regression into old behaviors and habits, remember that your good work up until that point has not been wasted. You do not have to start all over again. Not only will you be stronger, but you can learn from the experience so far and begin where you left off.

Motivated by compelling reasons for change, as well as by a global and inner understanding, by stopping the controllers and focusing on forgiveness of self and others, we are all capable of reaching our optimal level of HHP.

And now that you have a fresh, clean slate, it's time to envision and welcome great HHP by developing your own HeLP.

> ### *Nothing to Fear*
>
> *The R.E.L.I.E.F. Technique can be used to manage and let go of your current fears. Fear and worry are energy and health draining emotions, and both have their roots in uncertainty and on focusing on negative things that* ***could*** *happen. Humans have few genuine primal fears as infants: fear of falling, fear of sudden approach, and fear of loud noise.[24] Most other fears are created by our IMP. If we had a crystal ball and knew that everything would be all right, that we and our loved ones would live happily to a ripe old age, we would have no need to waste our energies on fear or worry. Unfortunately, there is no crystal ball. The only way to overcome our fears is to be aware of our destructive instincts and control our IMP and to be in the moment, in the heartbeat of our lives. As FDR said, we have nothing to fear but fear itself.*

Step 5 Exercise: R.E.L.I.E.F. List

With the level of awareness you now have it's time to list all of the mental manipulators in your life. Follow the steps as described a few pages back in the R.E.L.I.E.F. technique instructions. Use the table on the next page to record the following:

- Any destructive messy memory, event, experience, IMP, or instinct, etc.

- Any emotion(s) that each of the above stirs up

- Any current destructive habit(s) you think arises from that event or emotion

- Reason(s) you continue your destructive habit (or note anything that comes to mind as you go through the process)

Sample R.E.L.I.E.F. List – Use blank table on next page for your own list.

Destructive Memory/Event/Experience/IMP/Instinct/Etc.	Resultant Emotion	Adds to Which Destructive Habit	Reason(s) I Continue Destructive Habit; Notes
Messy Memory I fell in a mud puddle when 6 and thought it was funny, so I laughed, but Dad was angry and kicked me in the butt; told him I hated him	Shame, guilt, fear, humiliation, revenge, hate, regret	Excessive alcohol and marijuana; yelling excessively at my kids.	Feel peaceful and happy when high; Note: I must be easier on my kids
IMP Sister taught me to ridicule or assault other cultures and different skin colors	Pride, disdain, hate, shame	Aggressive behavior toward strangers	Protection from attack by others; display of strength
Instinct Envy of friends and others I see with new possessions and having a seemingly exciting life	Envy, sadness, hate, disappointment	I exaggerate about my income, experiences. I push my mate to make more money.	That others will be envious of my life; that I am important
IMP Religious traditions taught me to believe in things that harmed me and others	Confusion, shame, hate, fear	Destructive thinking instead of constructive	Note: I must practice my religion on my own terms
Instinct and IMP I exploit people, deplete earth's resources to maximize company profit	Happiness, security, desire, demanding	As long as legal, I will profit as much as possible	Money, security; everyone else does it; Note: find better way
Etc.	Etc.	Etc.	Etc.
(Blanket Statement) Any other destructive event, IMP, experience, or instinct	Any destructive emotion	Any destructive habit	Any reasons I continue destructive habit

When you have finished recording the *messy stuff,* continue from number 8, on page 141, until you complete the R.E.L.I.E.F. exercise. Congratulations on coming this far!

Step 5 Exercise: R.E.L.I.E.F. List – See Step 5 instructions on page 139.

Note: Copy this blank table for additional use.

Destructive Memory/Event/Experience/IMP/Instinct/Etc.	Resultant Emotion	Adds to Which Destructive Habit	Reason(s) I Continue Destructive Habit; Notes

Step 6: Develop Your HeLP

10

*Thought is the sculptor who can create
the person you want to be.*
—Henry David Thoreau

*If you plan on being anything less than you are
capable of being,
you will probably be unhappy all the days of your life.*
—Abraham Maslow

*The soul should always stand ajar,
ready to welcome the ecstatic experience.*
—Emily Dickinson

Your current level of HHP and where you would like it to be will be different than that of other people. For many people, setting out on the road to HealthyIsm will be like starting over and building a brand new life, a life of maintaining or welcoming greater health, happiness, and prosperity in all realms of their lives. For others, it will be more about tweaking areas of their lives that are not supporting their healthy evolution.

Regardless of where you started, you've already come a long way. You have identified what HealthyIsm is. You've learned what it means to be an Unhealthyolic and have asked yourself if you are one. You've also asked yourself if you can become healthier and have narrowed down your compelling reason to change.

In Steps 1 and 2 you became aware of your IMP and of the world around you. In Steps 3 and 4 you reviewed your life and identified problem areas. And in Step 5 you found ways to relieve yourself of any control these messy areas have over you and your life.

Now that you have a clean slate—an empty glass that you can fill with HealthyIsm—you need a well-thought-out plan that will turn confusion into clarity about how to welcome health, happiness, and prosperity. HealthyIsts realize that, unless a plan is already in place, they will need to set goals and design one that will help them welcome, calmly and kindly, a greater level of HHP. Your next step, then, is to develop your own personalized HealthyIsm Life Plan, or HeLP, that identifies all the angles and goals that will help you take one calm, kind, and bold step at a time toward a healthier, happier, and more prosperous lifestyle.

In Step 6, you will review what you learned in Step 2 about *your truth* to reprogram your IMP and develop your HealthyIsm Life Plan. To begin, you must first ask yourself, *What does an HHP life look like for me?* and then set goals to get yourself there. If you can already answer that question without hesitation, good for you! But if you're still unsure, go back to the statements in Step 2 to help you articulate your own goals.

For example, a person welcoming an HHP lifestyle may phrase his goals like this:

- To have inner awareness of my mind and how it controls me, and outer awareness of what's happening in the world

- To do healthy things like providing nutritious, healthy material to the body, mind, and soul and, at the same time, to be the protector of my body by keeping unhealthy things away or at least at a minimum

- To develop and maintain healthy relationships

- To acquire calmly, kindly, and fairly, and to maintain the resources that will support a healthy life for me and many others

Setting these goals is a crucial step, because they will be your lighthouse and help you set a clear direction for your thoughts and actions. They will help you develop supporting values, belief systems, and intentions so that you can truly be in charge of your IMP.

CHAPTER 10. STEP 6: DEVELOP YOUR HELP

HeLP: The HealthyIsm Life Plan

Back in Step 2 you analyzed and rated a series of statements that helped you pinpoint the current truth and reality of many aspects of your HHP. Now is the time to review the four distinct requirements of a constructive life and expand on its content in order to develop your HHP muscle. Just as your body will get stronger if you exercise, continually practicing the aspects that you develop in your HeLP will make them stronger.

Use the ideas here as a base to build your own HeLP—one that is right for you *at this time*. Once you have a taste of freedom from your Unhealthyolic habits—and start looking and feeling better because of your new habits—you may be inspired to keep pushing forward. You might also find that stopping one habit creates a domino effect on other habits. The same goes for starting healthy habits: once you master one healthy habit, others may fall into place almost effortlessly. And, of course, the big goal of the HeLP is to be totally aware of and to take control of your thoughts and actions so that you can be what you are capable of and create positive habits that will welcome HHP into your life.[25]

The essence of the draft plan laid out below is that, in order to attain greater HHP, we must optimally integrate all aspects of what it takes to have basic HHP. The basics can be had by using what we *know right now* about basic requirements of a constructive life, through rational thinking and scientific evidence. It also includes using the weird and wonderful stuff of spiritual and intuitive insights. Whether we *know* these insights to be true or not doesn't matter, because simply being open to them will help bring greater HHP to all.

The HeLP is divided into the four distinct requirements of a constructive life—called affirmations—that center around awareness, wellness, relationships, and resources. For each section, you will identify problem areas and develop a list of goals to welcome in that will support greater HHP in your life. You should also write down at least one action that will help you achieve each goal. Using the chart at the end of this chapter as a template, record these goals and actions in a journal, or on the computer—wherever is most useful for you.

Each affirmation is expanded upon below, with examples of the types of goals you might aim for in each section of your HeLP. Welcoming in these goals will ultimately reduce bad stress in your life, while moving away from them will increase bad stress. For example, in Silver Linings, if you are aware that something good always comes from something bad, then you will have less stress when something bad does occur.

Remember that the following HeLP is only a guide and not a definitive plan. Rather, it's a flex-

---

A Note about HeLP

Some of the information in this life plan may come across as idealistic. But we humans now have the power to make the changes necessary to welcome these so-called ideals. We are aware of our destructiveness, our own personal sickness, the sickness of humanity, and the unhealthy state of our earth. It's time to do the kind, calm, healthy, happy, and peacefully prosperous thing through calm critical thinking, focusing on the "I," applying the wisdom of past experiences, being mature, listening to our intuitive feelings, and working together to heal ourselves and the world.

ible draft on what it takes to be healthy, happy, and prosperous, and is meant to point you in the right direction and give you the tools to reach your destination. Some of the components may resonate with you; others may turn you off. Pick the ones that will help you not only break unhealthy habits but embrace your new "planned" ones.

The commonality behind all the following affirmations is that each one is about helping or supporting self and/or others to have a healthier, more constructive life.

Use this guide as a jumping-off point for creating your own unique HeLP. In the end, the exact components you come up with are secondary—what really matters is that, in developing your plan, you keep asking yourself the simple question: *Is this thought, action, habit, or goal supportive (or at least neutral) to me, others, and/or the earth, and does it ultimately welcome a calm and kind, healthy, happy, and prosperous evolution?*

Let's get started!

Affirmation 1: I Am Calmly Aware

The basis of your HeLP is to be aware of what's going on in the immediate environment of your body, mind, and soul, and in the world as a whole. Here are some awareness-related goals that will strengthen your chances of living a constructive life:

1. **Present moment.** I am calmly aware of this never-ending, exact moment where the future meets the past and of everything going on inside and around me. I am aware of my lungs, heart, and body; the visual surroundings,

smells, and sounds near and far; the "energy" emitted by others; the presence of an animal, tree, or lamppost; and the earth below and the universe above.

> √ Presence, living in the moment, helps you calm the mind, which often spends too much time regretting the past and fearing or desiring something in the future.

2. **Hidden agendas.** I am calmly aware of how others' agendas, sometimes hidden, sometimes unintended, are controlling the masses through various means like the media, religion, and our educational system. I am aware of the possibility that some of what I perceive to be true in our modern world may have been originally constructed by a few people who were acting within their own IMP and destructive instincts.

> √ That doesn't mean that you should mistrust anyone, only that you should investigate anything that could have a dramatic effect on your HHP.

3. **My IMP and its control over me.** I am calmly aware of my inner mental programming (IMP) and how it controls my life. I am conscious that my IMP influences the choices I make each day and the negative effects they may have. I am aware that my thoughts, the choices I make, and the actions I take co-create my reality with my reaction to the choices and actions of others and all acts of nature. I am aware that my IMP decides what is of value to and a priority for me, and that these values guide my every decision in life.

✓ Whatever you see in your life, from the shape and health of your body to the life you live, is largely influenced by the thoughts you think and your subsequent actions or reactions.

4. **Food and its effect on my mental chemistry.** I am calmly aware that what I ingest into my body affects my mind chemically and that there is a direct relationship between the foods I eat and the thoughts I think.

✓ A clear, sophisticated mental system is made up of neural pathways that are formed either by repetitive thoughts and actions or the foods you consume; for example, too much garbage "food" will lead to an unhealthy mental system.

5. **Food and its effect on my physical chemistry.** I am calmly aware that the food I ingest also affects my level of physical energy and is a key factor to being healthy.

✓ Eating a diet largely made up of whole, unprocessed, living foods that are raw or almost raw, low-gluten or gluten-free, and low-sugar or sugar-free—which means mostly fresh vegetables, sprouted nuts and seeds, some ripe fruits, some sprouted grains and perhaps for some people the occasional intake of a kindly cultivated organic animal protein—will likely keep you in your best health and have you jumping with energy. Eating excessive, isolated, cooked, and processed foods like burgers, fries, and soda may give you immediate pleasure, but they are sure to cause an energy crash, not to mention long-term mental and physical ill effects.

6. **Physical messages.** I recognize, acknowledge, and am calmly aware of the messages my body sends me.

√ The body is an amazing, complex machine with a built-in way to deliver messages about your current physical health. For example, a chronic inflamed toe with the medical label of "gout" is your body's way of telling you that there may be inflammation forming in other parts of the body, such as in the digestive system, and that something has to change.

7. **Being in tune with my meals.** I am calmly aware of and focused on my food *as I eat,* including the types of food and the quantities I am consuming.

√ Infants and animals are completely in the moment and focus intently on their food when they eat. As humans age, however, we are trained to look away from our food—either to speak to

A "Prayer" to My Food

Dear Food,

I acknowledge that you are a source of nutrients from God/ Universal Spirit/Nature, and I thank you for the life you have lived, the love you have given mother earth, and the love that you are giving me now. Your sacrifice to me is not in vain. I will assimilate your nutrients and essence into my body and move forward in the world to do good things. With much gratitude, Amen.[26]

another person, to read, or to watch TV—without giving it a second thought. This one goal alone—to truly be aware of the meal that you are assimilating into your flesh and bones by recognizing it as a gift and a life force full of nutrients, and by being in the moment with it by looking at it, smelling it, tasting it, and hearing it crunch—could transform your whole life! You may find yourself eating less and feeling happier and healthier.[27]

8. **Higher source.** I am calmly aware of my connection to a higher source, be it God or Universal Spirit or *something,* and feel connected to a state of oneness, a place that empowers me and gives me additional strength to stop my destructive habits. I regard my body as a temple that houses my soul, which is itself a droplet of God/Universal Spirit.

   √ If spiritual ideas don't resonate with you, try to regard yourself as a creation of a *physical* higher source called mother earth; we are all built with her raw materials—"from the earth we came, to the earth we go."

9. **General evolutionary purpose.** I am calmly aware of my "general evolutionary purpose" as a human, which is to adapt to and participate in the evolutionary process itself.

   √ Everything is evolving: the earth, plants, animals, and humans. Humans have not only evolved in our physical makeup but also in our knowledge of the world and the way things work. We are also evolving spiritually by being more aware of our connection to each other and to God/Universal Spirit. We are more aware that we are all connected as sensors, as receivers of "reality," as conscious tentacles of God/Universal Spirit, and as living mirrors bouncing back to God/Universal Spirit a reflection of the immense wonder of all existence. Where evolution will take us no one knows, but if we calmly and constructively work together to adapt to changes we are witnessing and participate in the evolutionary process in a conscious, healthy, aware way, it can only be a good thing. Being a part of the general evolutionary process will facilitate feelings of love, peace, and happiness.[28]

10. **Specific personal purpose.** Within my general evolutionary purpose, I have found and am calmly aware of my specific personal purpose.

    √ Knowing your purpose will help you ease your way into a healthy, happy, and prosperous life. Perhaps your specific purpose is to be a leader, or a follower, or to raise a child who becomes an inventor who creates a simple device that provides inexpensive, clean energy. It seems that all fulfilling life purposes have to do with helping others (including people, plants, and animals) either directly or indirectly. One way to find your life purpose is to ask the question: "If I had all the time in the world, and all my needs were met, what one thing could I do for another that would, at the same time, make me feel great?" Keep that question in front of you at all times and make it the last thing you read before you go to sleep. For more on finding your specific personal purpose, go to HealthyIsm.com.

11. **Direction.** I have created and am calmly aware of my vision and my direction in life.

   √ Knowing your specific purpose in life will go a long way in pointing you in the right direction. For example, if your specific purpose is to help people and the planet to be healthy, your direction might be to become an organic farmer who provides good food without harming the earth. In the same manner, you might become a healer to help the injured or sick or a business person to provide constructive, or at least neutral, services or products to humanity.

12. **No fear of death.** I am calmly aware of the death of the physical body as a natural process of life and know that it is not to be feared.

   √ There is a time to be born and a time to die. Yes, you must preserve and extend life as much as naturally possible (which can be done by practicing Healthy-Ism) and protect yourself from needless early departure from this great earth. But even if someone's life is tragically cut short, recognize that it was not in vain, because every person's life fits beautifully into the larger designs called the web of life and the cycle of life. And as religions and spiritual gurus teach, and as people who have had a near-death experience recount, there likely is a beautiful existence of peace, love, oneness, and enlightenment beyond our "living" days. After death we reconnect through awareness with God/Universal Spirit, like a branch would wake up and realize its connection to the tree. That's not to say that natural mourning and primal yearning for a deceased person aren't healthy, normal emotions; only that a prolonged state of depression in which a survivor is unable to function is neither healthy nor necessary. Even the first four stages of grieving—denial, anger, bargaining, and depression—can be overblown by your IMP. It's only in the fifth stage, acceptance, that we regain control. Continuous sadness can be a magnification of your IMP (which is partially programmed by society's conditioned denial of death) creating a thinking process that supports a "life is unfair, I'm so sad, I can't go on" state. It may be normal and healthy to be in that condition for a short time as a reaction to a death, but it is not healthy to live there forever. We may not see it initially, but immense sadness can act as a contrast to and enhance good times of health and happiness. On the other side of the same coin of sadness is its raw form - immense love. But one must tread these waters of raw sadness carefully so as not to be consumed. For example if a child is taken from his parents by a premature death, some people may cease to function for some time, or even forever, because of that primal sadness that is magnified by the IMP. But there are many examples of others who are able not only to control the IMP and move on from their primal sadness, but also to evolve to a higher level of consciousness and expand on their immense love of that child by creating everlasting memorials in the form of scholarships or charities in that child's name—and they do it with a smile of bittersweet love. Your human body is mortal. Your soul is immortal. The material that makes up your body, used and recycled since the beginning of time to construct all things, from rocks and plants to planets and humans, is also immortal. Yes, perhaps be concerned about the pain and suffering that may accompany death, but do not fear death. Fear of death in itself destroys *life;* no need to die twice.[29]

13. **Destructive instincts.** I am calmly aware of my instincts and that some of them may be destructive.

   √ Our beautiful bodies developed powerful instincts as a tool for survival in the harsh world of our ancestors. For example, instinctually we tend to freeze, flee quickly, or fight with fierce energy when faced with danger like a nasty, hungry animal. Our bodies create that extra energy to run or battle by activating the sympathetic nervous system, which is designed to stop unnecessary bodily functions like salivation, urination, and digestion. In our current society, survival instincts of the past have become unconsciously destructive to our lives. Most of us are in a constant fight-or-flight-or-freeze situation, faced with our modern "nasty animals" of a stressful job, dealing with traffic, shouting at our kids, facing an irate person lost in their IMP, trying to keep up with the Joneses, or just taking in the constant stream of bad news that the media gives us. The goal is to be aware of and control any urges that cause us to do the destructive things that we do. (See Chapter 5 for a review of destructive instincts.)

14. Rhythm. I am calmly aware of the daily, monthly, and yearly rhythm of my body and of the environment.

√ If you are a night owl, perhaps it's because your ancestors lived in a time zone five hours apart from yours. The rhythm of the seasons may cause you to need different nutrients. For example, if you are a meat eater, you'll want to consume sufficient amounts of meat in the winter when your body needs it, and very little, if any, in the summer. The rhythm of a woman's monthly cycle may also dictate the kind of food that makes her feel her best.

15. Silver linings. I am calmly aware that good things can often come from bad things.

√ The world is full of stories of people who have faced terrible situations only to find that, in the long run, their lives changed for the better. In my own life, for example, I contemplated suicide the night before I faced a lengthy sentence for a drug conviction. The short story is that, 16 years later, through constructive living, forgiving myself and others, finding the good in the bad, and the synchronicity of meeting various people in my life journey, my life is filled with goodness. Look for the silver lining; if you don't see it right away, just give it a little more time.

16. Global shift in consciousness. I am calmly aware that, collectively and individually, humans are evolving consciously to an understanding that we are much more than our bodies and that we are all part of a larger whole.

√ There are a growing number of aware people on the earth who are realizing the interconnectivity of all things and are looking for ways to be completely and collectively constructive, as opposed to continuing the destructive thoughts and actions that we give in to now.

HeLP Affirmation 2: I Am Well in Body, Mind, and Soul

As a maturing part of this organism called humanity, we must all give the physical, mental, and spiritual components of our bodies and beings the supporting material they need to stay strong. You need to develop habits that keep the physical body healthy by using it, providing it with proper nutrition, and keeping toxins at bay. You need habits that keep the mind healthy by exercising it, cleansing it of negative thoughts, and feeding it with emotional attentiveness and helpful knowledge. And you need habits that keep your spirit strong by *listening* to your intuition, being present, and finding time to play, laugh, and meditate or pray regularly. For those who are not into the spiritual stuff, that's okay; call it contemplating or focusing, or just skip it and build on the rest.

> ### The Evolving Soul
>
> *The soul can be looked at as a holographic drop of the eternal ocean of infinite Source power. It is a spark of Universal Spirit, Nature, or God that provides living energy to our bodies. Like a pacemaker without a battery, a body without a soul-spark is lifeless.*
>
> *Source power, intending to create and evolve, to explore and experience its vastness of Omni-self through all sensing organisms, co-creates our reality by guiding our soul-spark through intuition and emotions. If we welcome the guidance, Source power inspires our thinking and ultimately evolves our reality*
>
> *French philosopher Pierre Teilhard de Chardin said that we are heading for an "omega point," meaning that the human body appears to be evolving to a maximum level of complexity and consciousness.*
>
> *Our souls are also evolving, awakening the minds of all humans to their integral connection to source power and to each other. With maturing souls, we are becoming less inclined to defend destructive positions of our instincts and programmed minds and instead welcome all that is good.*

Here are some goals related to being well in body and mind and soul:

1. **Multi-functional exercise.** I physically use my body for the many functions for which it was designed and intended, such as pushing, pulling, running, walking, climbing, squatting, twisting, lifting, and throwing.

√ If you have a physical job like farming or construction, you most likely do all these things already. If you have a sedentary profession, then exercising with these motions in mind will keep your body fit. (See Appendix A and HealthyIsm.com for more information on exercise.)

2. **Just enough exercise.** I give my body enough exercise to keep it fit but not enough to harm it.

√ Both too much and too little exercise will have a negative effect on the body. Over-exercising can wear out your joints, break down muscle, weaken the immune system, and leave you tired. Too little exercise speaks for itself—use it or lose it! Not only will sufficient exercise keep your muscles intact, it will also increase your energy, aid in digestion, and move fluids through your system.

3. **Proper fuel.** I give my body and mind the proper fuel they need to get and stay healthy.

√ Whether you are a meat eater or a vegetarian, eating lots of nutrient-dense foods like vegetables—the rawer the better—is absolutely key to good health. Deciding whether to be vegetarian, vegan, or omnivorous really depends on your body type (which is determined by your genetic makeup) and what's going on in your life. For example, during a hot season, meat eaters likely need less or no meat; if you are female and menstruating, you may need to eat meat to build your iron stores, even if you are genetically a vegetarian. If you are not getting the nutrients in the food that you eat, then supplementation through minerals and vitamins may be necessary. Also make sure you are drinking the proper amount of water. Some of your water intake can be substituted with freshly squeezed vegetable juice. (See HealthyIsm.com for more information on what to eat, supplementation, water intake, and how to determine your body makeup.)

4. **Just enough fuel.** I give my body enough fuel to keep it fit but not enough to harm it.

   √ For those of us who are part of the privileged society, we simply eat too much food. Getting the proper fuel is important, but so is making sure you don't take in too much. You'll find that not only can you function on much less, but that you'll feel more energized and mentally clearer.

5. **Just enough sunshine.** I get enough daily sunshine but not enough to cause harm.

   √ Just as plants require sunshine for photosynthesis, humans require regular sunshine on the majority of the body at the right time of day to boost mood, produce vital vitamin D, and much more. The fear of the sun that we as a society have embraced may be causing us more harm than good. A lot of recent research suggests that we need more sun not less. Go to HealthyIsm.com for more information on sunshine and the benefits of vitamin D.

6. **Toxin free.** I do what I can to control the toxins in my body.

  √ In today's world, it is virtually impossible to keep the toxins out of our bodies. One way to control toxins is to keep your eliminatory systems working properly and watch what you put into your mouth. Besides providing a higher nutrient content, going as organic as possible and drinking an appropriate amount of water will at least help keep commercial, toxin-laden foods out of your system.[31]

7. **Treat control.** I limit my intake of treats and control my IMP when it has the urge to indulge.

  √ The endorphins released and the smile you get when you have a cookie or a glass of wine or a joint may have a place in your health and happiness. But when you find the treat consuming you instead of you consuming it, it's time to control those indulgences. The best bet is to stay completely away from stimulants, but if you do want to include them in your life, find a schedule for them—once a week, once a month, once a year, once a decade. Knowing that you are still allowed to have something that you like may be a way to keep you smiling between treats! And as time goes by, the desire for the treats may become less and less.

8. **Mental-robics.** I keep my mind healthy, crisp, and clear by challenging it on a daily basis through problem solving, creative pursuits, and challenging my memory.

- √ Feed your mind with health-supporting information, and keep pessimistic news in check. Read in areas of your interest and also in areas you don't care much about. Do something different daily to build new neurons. Knit something if you're a sports jock; try a sport you've never played if you're a knitter. Practice visualizing—that is, concentrating on images in your mind with as much detail as possible so that you imagine a clear picture with sounds, smells, and tastes. These types of exercises will keep the mind sharp and well-rounded. (See HealthyIsm.com for a list of mental exercises.)

9. **Support a positive mental state.** I feed my mind with "good" things.

- √ For a cheerful, optimistic, and constructive mental state, find and feed your mind constructive information, news, and ideas like stories about acts of goodness done by others, the best foods, the best way to live a constructive life, the best exercises, and ideas for building abundance.

Join a Brief, Twice-Daily Global Meditation, Prayer, or Focus

The practice of HealthyIsm encourages all people, no matter where they are in the world or from what religious, cultural, or other background, to jointly pause momentarily, for once or both of the two synchronized daily times, to meditate, pray, or focus (MPF) on any or all of the following:
- *global connection through a spiritual oneness sense and/or an awareness of the physically shared living earth below their feet*
- *a vision of a healthy I and healthy world*
- *the pulse of the present moment*
- *and/or simply good feelings*

This global MPF, this collective constructively conscious brain power, is coordinated to two fixed daily times of noon and midnight GMT (Greenwich Mean Time). The goal is to be globally aware, cooperative, and constructive.

When you are MPF-ing, be aware of others doing the same with you at the same time. Also, physically or mentally, place one hand over your brain, representing control of IMP and instincts, and one hand over your heart, representing acting with love. If one of the times falls during your sleep, don't worry; just join the world at the other fixed time—but tell yourself as you fall asleep that you will be participating in your slumber. Wherever and whoever you are, join the global tribe daily for at least one of those two pauses. Once you find yourself participating on a regular basis, the next step is to make the global connected mindset a constant part of your day. Also spread the word and encourage others to participate in this daily global MPF. Go to HealthyIsm. com for details and the exact daily times in your region.

10. Meditate, pray, or focus often. I strengthen my spiritual awareness of and connection to Universal Spirit/God and/or others and to the earth below my feet by meditating, praying, or focusing (MPF) regularly.

√ Take the time to relieve your mind of the endless mental chatter and stresses of daily living, become aware of your connection to all things, and just be flesh and bones observing what is. As bio-bots (biological robots) of a time-programmed world, our minds naturally race from analyzing the past to planning the future. It's *time* to get away from *time* and be one with the flow of all things as if you are a droplet in an ocean of reality. Pick one point of focus like a plant, a candle flame, your child, a rock, or your breathing. Using your breath is a fabulous way to relax and be with the moment. Don't think about it; just be with it. If your mind wanders, tell yourself that's okay and bring it back to the object of focus. Or just be an observer of your wandering mind. The goal is to be present with the moment without worrying about the future or revisiting the past. Just be with everything that exists around you at this exact moment, and then this exact moment, and then…and so on. Also be aware of the shared, living, evolving earth below your feet as a commonality between all people. See yourself growing out of the earth like a blade of grass, connected in the lawn of humanity. You may find a deep sense of unity and inner peace that is beyond any thought. You might have already experienced such moments when you caught a peaceful nap on a beautiful, stress-free spring day or lovingly stretched out without thought beside your newborn baby. During your MPF time you can instead or also think of anything that gives you those feelings, like an enjoyable hobby, a cookie, a walk on the beach, loving sex, a stroll through the forest, relaxing on a comfy couch, or an adoring and kind grandparent. The idea is to create a good vibe, a feeling of love, happiness, or peace. Take a deep, slow breath in.... (See HealthyIsm.com for a recorded MPF session.)

11. **Sleepy time.** I understand how much sleep my body needs and ensure that I get it.

    √ Our bodies were hormonally designed to go to sleep soon after sunset and to awaken soon after sunrise. Many of us go to bed late and still get up early for our daily responsibilities. It's so important to know how much rest your body needs and to be vigilant about your down time! (See HealthyIsm.com for tips and information on sleep.)

12. **Quiet rest.** I give my body, mind, and soul the quiet and rest they need to digest and assimilate all the good stuff that I am giving them.

    √ In addition to your sleep time, take time on a daily basis, even for just a few minutes, to be by yourself and feel your body, the earth below, and the universe in you and outside of you. Feel your muscles and *mind* relax.

13. **Laugh, dance, sing, and play.** I take the time to honor

the child within and to laugh, dance, sing, and play!

√ If you watch a child who has not yet learned to "act like an adult," you'll see him do these four things and more all day long. Laughing, dancing, singing, and playing are innate and pure activities—and when you ensure that they are a regular part of your daily routine, they will bring you fuel for happiness. Have a sense of humor, be silly, dance to your favorite song or a tune in your head, sing along or make up your own song, and play with no rules attached. Feel your energy soar.

14. **Emotional health.** I am in tune with my emotions, where they are coming from, and what messages they are delivering to me.

√ Pure, innate emotions are like a communication system that sends messages from Universal Spirit/God into your mind. Your emotions not only guide your direction but also help you know what to do for others. If you see an old person in need of help and feel empathy and a need to act, it's Universal Spirit/God giving you direction and guidance. In this way, the spirit directs the emotions to influence the mind to direct the body. If you feel angry, frustrated, hateful, or fearful, something in your life has to change, whether it be the thoughts you're thinking or the direction you're going in. If you always feel happy, optimistic, loving, and peaceful, then just keep doing what you're doing… you are likely on the right path. (See HealthyIsm.com for more information on emotional health.)

HeLP Affirmation 3: I Nurture My Relationships

Your overall goal in this area is to develop a network of healthy, trusting, truthful, forgiving, and loving relationships with yourself and others. The idea is to build and maintain a community of relations; it's healthy for the I and healthy for the world. With calm awareness, trust others and yourself to do the HealthyIsm thing instead of wasting energy on distrust. Treat others as if they were part of yourself. Be truthful; there is no higher power than truth, so see and say the truth whenever possible. Always forgive; forgiveness is based in love. If someone tells you or you tell yourself the truth about a given situation that requires forgiveness, then forgive and move on. Be equally loving to yourself and others with the same profound, pure love you find between a mother and child.

One way to motivate yourself to do so is to recognize that all life is fundamentally interconnected and interdependent—what I do to you, I do to myself; what I do to myself, I do to you. And that's why HealthyIsm is about focusing on the I. Healthy I, healthier relationships.

Consider these relationship goals as you develop your HealthyIsm Life Plan:

1. Love myself. I strengthen and maintain the number-one relationship in my life—my relationship with myself.

> √ This is your most important and foundational relationship. Be easy on yourself for all the Unhealthyolic things you have done to others and to yourself. You

can also be easy on yourself by forgiving any harm that others have done to you. Remember that holding on to the hate or anger caused by the stupidity of someone else is like swallowing poison and expecting the other person to die—it doesn't bother the other person a bit, and you're the only one to suffer.

2. My "true" love. I strengthen and maintain a meaningful relationship with my significant other.

√ A "true love" relationship may be tough, but oh, so rewarding! Having a compatible (yet different enough to keep things spicy) significant other with whom to share life's experiences, be sexually and lovingly intimate, raise a family, and build a legacy just magnifies the human experience and makes it that much better. Practice patience and tolerance when it comes to the unhealthy habits of your love, and continue to improve the bond by improving yourself. Healthy I, healthy relationship.

3. Love my coworker. I develop healthy and mutually beneficial relationships with my coworkers and colleagues.

√ We often spend more time with the people at work than we do with our own families, so having a "loving" relationship with your coworkers, employees, or boss will make your days much easier. Strive to be as compassionate, loving, and cooperative as possible, and recognize that they are also human beings and Unhealthyolics who are operating to the best of their abilities. Learn to forgive and accept them as they are and continue to work on the one person you know best—you! As you begin to embrace a life of Healthy-Ism, your coworkers will see and be inspired by the change in the way you think and act.

4. **Love my family.** I strengthen and maintain my relationships with members of my immediate and extended family.

   √ All the people of this great planet are part of one large family, but the people you get to practice "familyship" with are closest to you and know you best—and therefore deserve your special attention. After all, what you practice at home is reflected in how you and your family act and react in the world. If your children aren't turning out the way you'd like, remember that they have learned their way of being mostly from you. They are the fruit of the tree (you) from which they fell. Instead of lecturing them about their behavior, show by example. Show them how to be easy, forgiving, and loving with yourself and others. When you mess up with them, own up to it with a smile, forgive yourself, and keep the momentum going toward a life of HealthyIsm.

5. **Love earth and all its nature.** I love, honor, and respect the earth by developing healthy habits.

   √ As mentioned throughout this book, having a loving, respectful relationship with the mother of us all, mother earth and all its nature, will be a tremendous help to you as you strive to stop unhealthy habits and embrace a healthy lifestyle. How do you best help the earth? By treating yourself with the utmost respect. Think of your body as another part of the earth (like the rest of the plants and animals), a diverse mini-earth with its own ecosystems of different parts, organs, and chemicals—and treat all parts of the earth, your body included, with great respect and love.

6. **Love Universal Spirit/God.** I strengthen and maintain my relationship to my spiritual self through my relationship with Universal Spirit/God.

√ The greatest relationship of all lies beyond and within ourselves, others, and the earth; it is the one we have with Universal Spirit/God. Even without proof, many people believe that there is something larger than us that has the power to keep order and give life to everything in the universe, from the human body to the pinecone. Having a relationship with or acknowledging Universal Spirit/God—even if you believe it to be a "placebo"—can be truly empowering. We know that the power of the mind can create miracles, so why not believe in and co-participate with an omnipresent energy or being that may be both larger than you and reside within you?

7. **Love my neighbor, near and far.** I know, support, and love my neighbors both locally and globally.

√ Don't worry if your local neighbors are not the type to mingle—it's enough to be open to any possible interaction. Offer small acts of kindness without looking for anything in return, like stopping by your neighbors' with a holiday gift, cleaning the snow from their driveway, or picking up a piece of trash from their property. You may even simply offer a smile. Approach everyone in your local community with the same attitude and extend that attitude to the rest of the world. Offer support in whatever way you can and treat everyone as part of a large, precious family.

8. Charity partnership. I give portions of my time, money, or support to charitable causes.

√ Offering any kind of support to those in need is as good a medicine for you as it is for the recipient. You can start small by looking for local volunteer opportunities in your area such as reading to a blind person, taking a dog for a walk at an animal shelter, participating in a fundraiser, or visiting a senior at a long-term care facility. Or you can take on a larger project like building and staffing an emergency shelter. Try it—the people you help will appreciate it, and you'll love it! See Chapter 14 for more ideas on supporting others.

HeLP Affirmation 4: I Build and Maintain Resources

You must develop peacefully and acquire fairly the tools, resources, and assets that will help you welcome and maintain a life of HealthyIsm. If you had to build a house, you'd find that the more resources and materials you had available, the better the quality of the structure and the faster you could complete it. Your HHP is the same way: you can use your basic program and tools to get along very nicely and live healthily to a ripe old age—but with better resources and better tools, you'll break unhealthy habits faster and more easily and be able to embrace an HHP lifestyle sooner. The important thing to remember is no excuses. Use what you have to build and maintain a supply of resources, and keep moving forward.

Read through the different types of resources and their related goals below to help you form your own resource goals for your Plan:

1. **My thoughts.** I use my biggest resource of all—my thoughts—to start from a place of gratitude and to create a positive reality.

    √ Practice focused, grateful, positive thoughts on a daily basis: concentrate on what you want in life, not on what you don't want. As you identified in the Awareness section, many other people and institutions have been responsible for creating your reality. Your schooling, parents, culture, religion, and the outside input you receive from various media largely dictate the way you think and, as a result, what becomes your reality. As you gain more control over your IMP and instincts and begin to think for your optimal evolution, welcoming in the beneficial aspects of your programming such as the ancient wisdom of your culture, you will have a better chance of creating a life as you choose. If you are reading this book, then it is very likely that you are on your way to creating a life full of healthiness, happiness, and prosperity.

2. **Questions.** I ask myself focused, positive questions that, in finding the answers, help me welcome great HHP.

   √ This resource alone could be all you need to push your HeLP toward great success. Pose your questions in terms of what you want instead of what you don't want. For example, instead of asking yourself, *How can I avoid being sick?*, you ask, *How do I become and stay healthy?* The simple question we often ask in HealthyIsm is: *Is this thought or action supportive (or at least neutral) to me, others, and/or the earth, and does it ultimately welcome a calm and kind, healthy, happy, and prosperous evolution? If not, what thought or action would be supportive?*

3. **Communication.** I regularly practice delivering my thoughts clearly to others and receiving information clearly and as intended by others.

   √ Unless you live as a hermit, effective communication skills are an essential resource. Ultimately we all speak the same language—the human language. We communicate through eye contact, facial expressions, sounds, hugs, intonations, intuition, appreciation, respect, handshakes, bows, and yes, actual spoken language. (See HealthyIsm.com for more information on communication.)

4. **Good health.** I continuously improve or maintain a healthy body.

   √ A strong, healthy body and mind gives you the energy

and clarity you need to achieve your goals in life. A sick body will only divert energy to the recovery process and slow you down. Just remember that th*ere are no excuses*—move forward from wherever you are, kindly and calmly at your own speed, and you'll see that living healthy will get easier over time.

5. **Intuition.** I recognize and trust my "gut feelings" about my choices and situations in life.

   √ Listening to what your "inner voice" tells you about your choices will help guide you toward a healthier life. It is said that we speak to Universal Spirit/God through prayer and meditation and that Universal Spirit/God speaks to us through intuition. When you "hear" yourself saying "this feels right" or, conversely, "there is something I don't like about this," make note of it and see what the outcome is. Knowing that your intuition is real and trusting what it says to you is a great resource.

6. **Support network.** I strive to build a network of family, friends, and community that I can rely on for support when I need it.

   √ Make connections with others at every opportunity. Offer support to others when they are in need, and be open to ask for support when the role is reversed. (See the Relationship section in this chapter for thoughts on developing and maintaining strong relationships. You can also visit HealthyIsm.com to link up with the HealthyIsm support network.)

7. **Wisdom.** I learn from my experiences and life lessons and use that knowledge as a source of wisdom and insight to make better decisions.

   √ You only need to touch a hot light bulb once to be wise enough not to do it again. Recalling knowledge you've gained through experiences and through lessons learned from others who share their wisdom with you will be an invaluable resource in your quest to live a healthy life.

8. **Talents.** I recognize and hone my own special talents.

   √ We all have different wiring and unique physical capabilities that make us able to do certain things better than others. Discover what those things are for yourself. Knowing that you have a knack for numbers, an artistic creativity, or natural leadership abilities will help you choose where and how to spend your energies and time.

9. **Jolly job.** I have found or am looking for a job or career that is challenging, interesting, and fulfilling—in short, a job I love.

   √ Until humans learn to share the earth's resources, it's a benefit to have a job, preferably one you love, to help acquire at least the basic necessities of life. For many people, finding that perfect job is easier said than done. Taking the time to understand and be aware of who you are and what you want in life will help steer you toward a profession or job that you'll look forward to every day, whether it be your own business or working for someone else. Working with people you like, enjoying the environment you're in, having ample vacation and recreation time, and being sufficiently paid will help you feel excitement each day as you engage professionally and will make for a healthier, happier, and more prosperous life. Be clear on how much time you want to dedicate to work so that it will not cause an imbalance in other areas of your HeLP. If you are currently working at a job you don't like, then the first thing to do is *change your attitude*. Go with the flow; try looking at your job as part of a larger, interconnected purpose. If you're a sweeper, know that your work helps others in your company focus and operate better in theirs. Once you've got that attitude of gratefulness and interconnectedness, start welcoming new job possibilities into your life.

10. **Productivity.** I am productive both professionally and personally.

√ There is no better feeling than setting out on a project and knowing that you can produce results effectively and efficiently. Be mindful that your productivity is constructive, and ensure that what you produce has positive (or at least neutral) effects on you, others, and the earth.

11. **Cash and assets.** I strive to build and use my financial resources wisely, responsibly, and knowledgably.

√ Cash in the bank, a piece of land to stand on, and other

assets can be used as leverage as you implement and maintain your HeLP. Welcome in being free of debt and investing wisely to build your cash reserve. Invest in environmentally and human-friendly tools, products, and services. Until the time humans can reasonably share all of earth's resources, find a way to buy land or property to constructively develop and nurture, and as a long-term investment.

12. **Getaway places.** I have welcomed into my life a place to regularly "get away from it all."

    √ Be it a cottage, a favorite bed and breakfast, a seasonal travel destination, a wellness retreat, a quiet spot in your home (yes, even the bathroom), or a grassy spot under a tree in a public park, use your getaway place as a point of decompression where you can close your eyes, reconnect with nature, and just be with yourself for a moment or two.

13. **Tools for daily life.** I have the tools and equipment I need to make my daily life run smoothly.

    √ Don't overlook the everyday items that can help you in your quest for optimal health, be it an environmentally friendly car, a computer, business equipment, or a wheelchair. Make sure you also have the tools you need—a hammer, a musical instrument, gardening tools, a paint brush, a pen and some paper—so that you can create your own "stuff," as we humans are so capable of doing.

14. **Willpower.** I develop and use my willpower as a resource for self-control.

    √ If you have trouble completing tasks or sticking to a plan, then you need to develop your willpower. Start small, then work your way up to larger goals. For example, if you want to lose weight, just say to yourself, "I will eat optimally for one day." The next day say, "I will eat optimally for two days," and so on. Then stick to it!

15. **Forgiveness.** I have it locked into my brain that all transgressions against me or against myself are ultimately to be forgiven—not necessarily forgotten, but definitely forgiven.

    √ Welcome forgetting about a transgression in a way that you don't worry about it anymore. The ability to forgive is one of the greatest assets you can have. Holding onto resentment is poisonous to our bodies, to our religions, to our nations, and to our world. Exercise forgiveness as you would any muscle and watch as your capacity to forgive gets stronger. Forgive huge things and small things. Forgive an abuser who has caused immense pain; forgive yourself for missing the exit on the highway. Remember that forgiveness means the freedom to fill your life with love and good things.

16. **Little or no clutter.** I continually get rid of clutter in my head, my closet, my house, my garage, my car, and my life.

√ With the exception of items of true sentimental value, the general rule is that anything you haven't used in a year (or a maximum of two) gets thrown on the "out" pile. Get rid of it! Every year, do a spring "kijiji cleaning"—www.kijiji.com is an items-for-sale website where you can list all your never-used stuff and rake in a little dough. Make space for positive change and allow new and improved stuff to flow in!

17. **The Internet.** I use the Internet to share and receive knowledge and to be globally connected.

√ The Internet has given humans the opportunity to communicate instantly with each other on a mass scale. With this resource, we can deliver messages, share knowledge, and offer tools, products, and services to the world.

18. **Stress.** I understand that a certain amount of stress is good for me.

√ What? Stress as a resource? Yes! Just as physical stress (exercise) helps your muscles develop, the right amount of stress in other areas of your life helps your body, mind, and soul develop. For example, the occasional stress of sadness or loneliness will strengthen your love "muscle"; the occasional short bout of the flu or common cold will stress and strengthen your immune system; the stress of physical labor will produce positive physical results; and the stress of studying will strengthen your mind.[32]

19. **Stress releasers.** I have developed healthy methods of releasing stress and controlling the stress levels in my life.

    √ When things get tough, many people retreat into unhealthy habits like drinking, overeating, or high-intensity exercise in an effort to relieve the stress—unaware, of course, that such behaviors produce more harmful stress! Find healthy alternatives for releasing stress in the difficult moments of your life. Meditation or quiet time, a very light workout/stretch, or listening to relaxing music will be more beneficial than getting high or going on a high-impact run.

20. **Truth.** I live a life of truth. I am a truthful person, because always coming from a place of truth not only resonates well with others but also energizes me and puts me in alignment with the universe.

    √ What a powerful resource! Truth will set you free to be healthy, happy, and prosperous. Truth may be painful but is ultimately a good pain. Dishonesty causes an imbalance in your system, but "coming clean"—living in truth—helps restore balance and peace in your life. And truthfulness makes your relationships easier and more fulfilling because people know they can trust you and are truthful with you in return. "Little white lies" may be sensible and necessary on occasion (for example, to protect someone who may not be ready or able to handle a particular truth), but whenever possible, simply tell the truth. Be especially truthful to yourself and know that it's okay to admit things to yourself (for example, that perhaps you've let your instincts and your IMP control you all your life, that you have sexual urges for a friend, that you are addicted to something, or that your religion may include some destructive weak points).

21. **Self-defense.** I have learned methods of defending myself in worst-case scenarios.

    √ Unfortunately, until all humanity wakes up to the destructive nature of the IMP, you'll need to know how to defend yourself in various ways. Of course, you are encouraged to go through life avoiding clashes of your IMP with that of others, but the reality is that in a world that has not fully embraced HealthyIsm, emergency situations do arise. Learn basic self-defense (including non-violent techniques), be aware of your surroundings, and make calm (not crazy!), careful choices when it comes to your personal safety.

22. **Sacrifice.** When and if I choose to do so, I allow the sacrifice of various aspects of my own health, happiness, and prosperity in order to help others positively evolve. I am aware that doing so ultimately helps me and the world.

    √ Parents sacrifice aspects of their lives all the time for the sake of their children, while people like Mother Teresa and Gandhi made extreme sacrifices for the betterment of others. The bottom line is that if someone is ready and willing to improve her life and requests your help, then sacrificing your finances, sleep, personal de-stress time, or exercise time to support her may be well worth the results. For example, if your loved one is sick and needs help, then obviously letting go of some of your sleep, meditation, and play time to take care of him/her is a worthy sacrifice. But be careful: if it's obvious that the other person is not serious about overcoming his or her Unhealthyolic habits, then sacrificing your own constructive life might not be the way to go.

23. Time. I use time as a resource for such pursuits as dedicating the time needed to create and maintain a healthy lifestyle.

√ As you set out to break destructive habits, you *may* find it difficult at first—but it will get easier over *time* for all the reasons laid out in this book. The more *time* you spend practicing living a healthy life, the better your chances of overcoming your old unhealthy habits. As you use time, be aware that it is a mental construct of the human mind as a means to organize our weird but wonderful world which in turn has immense control over our lives. Use it, but don't let it use you. Recognize when the ticking of the clock is causing you more sorrow then joy. Take a "time-break" and submerse yourself in nature for a day or three using only the beautiful rhythm of the day sun and night stars to balance your biological clock.

24. Earth. I recognize and respect mother earth as the great fragile resource it is.

√ A happy, healthy, prosperous life largely depends on mother earth, which supplies us with so many gifts. In addition to its obvious gifts of air, food, water, and shelter, the earth also offers such wonderful stuff as energy systems and eco-diversities. One thing you must learn to do is to ensure that the earth is *always* treated as a sustainable, fragile resource. Regardless of what you take from it, you must ensure that you have a positive, or at least neutral, effect. You must ensure that you are careful with other people, other animals, the forests, the oceans, soil usage, toxic chemicals, and nature's balance. Invest in and demand constructive tools, products, services, cheap and clean fuel sources, and organic, unprocessed foods.

25. **Peace.** I am peaceful with self and others as often as possible.

    √ When we are at peace with ourselves and with each other, we live more in an anabolic, parasympathetic state, which is a state of repair, regeneration, and rejuvenation. The world and humanity have been in the fearful, catabolic, fight-or-flight-or-freeze, sympathetic state for too long. Peace on earth and peace of mind will repair our earth and heal our bodies.

26. **Calculated risk.** I move outside of my safety zone and take occasional calculated risks.

    √ Most things we do involve some degree of risk: driving a car, snowboarding, starting a new business, interacting with people, or even sleeping in bed (your home could catch fire in the middle of the night). Taking calculated risks where you put the odds in your favor is the key. Taking a defensive driving course and making sure your vehicle is maintained, taking snowboarding lessons and always using a helmet, analyzing all parts of a business venture, being calmly aware of the people you interact with, and keeping your home fire-safe by maintaining smoke detectors and fire extinguishers will improve your odds of evolving safely. Having calculated risk as a resource also allows creativity to flow. New ideas, inventions, magical arts, and the like come from those who are willing to risk stepping outside the conventional norm.

27. **Choice:** the power to support and influence corporations and governments. I do what I can to ensure that companies and governments learn to live a life of HealthyIsm, including choosing where to vote or trade my dollars for tools, services, and products.

√ Individual private usage of our earth's resources only accounts for 25% of all consumption; the majority is being used by the "big guys and gals." As part of the greater group, you have the power to vote for governments that welcome a kind and calm HHP evolution and to support corporate services and products that do the same.

28. **My HealthyIsm Life Plan.** I have a clear vision of my goals and a concrete plan for welcoming them in.

√ Just as a roadmap helps you reach a specific destination more quickly and efficiently, so will having clear goals to welcome into your life. Think about your goals, then write them down (which you have done in this HeLP section), paint a picture, make them your screen saver, or do whatever you need to do to keep that vision in front of you. Don't worry if you have the "right" vision or not—as you move forward, it will become clearer and you can adjust accordingly. Some signs that tell you that you're welcoming the right things into your life are that you smile more, feel really good about yourself, have lots of energy, have improved your HHP, and see others following your example and bettering their own lives.

You should now have a good list of goals and actions for each HeLP affirmation. Don't overwhelm yourself in trying to make it all happen at once; just affirm to yourself that you are open to welcoming each part of your plan into your life at your own pace. Remember that this HeLP is only the author's consideration of what to welcome into his own life. Make this *your* plan, so if you have something to add or change, feel free to do so. (If you think others can benefit from your change or new idea, please let us know by visiting the HealthyIsm website forum and joining the "Modify the HealthyIsm Life Plan" thread.)

Pain and Suffering

Although the HeLP does not refer to pain or suffering, we do recognize that they are part of the human condition. If you are suffering or in pain—for example, you're living with a degenerative disease, having relationship or business problems, if you're a citizen of a corrupted or war torn country, or feeling depressed—then at the moment you may only be able to "be" with your pain and suffering and nothing else. But when you're ready and feel that it's time to move forward, to welcome better health, happiness, and/or prosperity, you can apply the contents of this book and use the HeLP as a starting point and a guide.

If you are of sound mind and are considering any major changes in your life (including undertaking this seven-step HealthyIsm program), be sure to discuss these changes beforehand with your primary, up-to-date health care provider.

Many of the components outlined in this HeLP can be expanded on immensely. For example, volumes of books have been written on the subject of being in the now, which we touch on only lightly in the Present Moment paragraph in the Awareness section. The focus of your personalized HeLP is on identifying what you would like to calmly and kindly welcome into your life in order to optimize and balance your life, and then doing what it takes and opening yourself to receive it.

Now that you have your HeLP and a clear vision of where you want to go, it's time to look at ways of making your life of HealthyIsm a reality. It's time to do what it takes and support your plan.

Step 6 Exercise: Create a HealthyIsm Life Plan

AFFIRMATION 1: I Am Calmly Aware		
Areas In Which To Increase Awareness	Goal	Action
Present moment	To be less in my head and more in the moment	Every time the kids are causing trouble, I will be aware of the beauty of all things going on around me and react calmly.

AFFIRMATION 2: I Am Well in Body, Mind, and Soul		
Areas in Which to Foster Wellness	Goal	Action
Multi-functional exercise	To use my body as it was designed	Start a sizeable and vigorous garden project in which I will use my whole body.

HealthyIsm: *Healthy I, Healthy World!*

AFFIRMATION 3: I Nurture My Relationships		
Areas To Nuture Relationships	Goal	Action
Love myself	*To strengthen my relationship with me!*	*Be easy on myself for anything that I do. Treat myself regularly to massages or other pleasant experiences.*

AFFIRMATION 4: I Build and Maintain Resources		
Areas To Build Or Maintain Resources	Goal	Action
My thoughts	*To use my thoughts as a resource to create a constructive reality*	*Feed my mind good things and shut off negative media.*

Step 7: Support Your HeLP

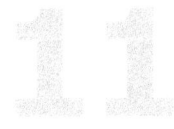

The gods help them that help themselves.
—Aesop

Fall seven times, stand up eight.
—Japanese Proverb

*When you come to the end of your rope,
tie a knot and hang on.*
—Franklin D. Roosevelt

Whew! Building health, happiness, and prosperity in your life may not be easy, but it will be incredibly rewarding. During your journey to HealthyIsm you may experience many obstacles and setbacks. The most important thing to remember is that it's okay! Just keep practicing; not only will you get used to your new lifestyle, but more and more people around you will become aware of the illusions that surround them and start living healthier lives as well. And as humanity evolves and becomes more informed, it's becoming "cool" (and easy) to think and act upon thoughts that support your constructive evolution.

Heal and Evolve

As a collective, we're becoming less and less unaware—or at least we now have the means to be aware through the instant interconnectivity of the "worldwide web" of life (and the ability to share lots of knowledge, fast). This means that by practicing a HealthyIsm lifestyle, seeing how well it works for you, and then sharing it with others, the earth and humanity may actually heal and evolve beyond the sickness and craziness that we are experiencing today. Your commitment to constructive consciousness, to a healthy *I,* means that you have chosen not to be ignorant or negligent and instead to contribute to the well-being of yourself, others, the earth, and beyond.

Remember that in the fairy tale *The Three Little Pigs,* the pig who put in the time and effort to build a strong brick house had a much better chance of withstanding the evil force of the wolf. Building a strong HeLP piece by piece—and then fortifying it with the suggestions presented in this chapter—will help you withstand the unhealthy forces of sickness, negative self-talk, negativity of others, toxic environments, people with hidden agendas, and more.

In Step 6, you worked really hard to draft your HealthyIsm Life Plan. You have done well so far and have gone from not knowing what was happening with your HHP to knowing what you want to welcome into your life. Your HeLP may be just a first draft not written in stone, but it will give you direction until you find a need to revise or improve it.

But now it's time to wipe the sweat from your brow and continue on. It's time to do whatever it takes to encourage a successful outcome. It's time to support your HeLP. The best approach for you will be different than for others. You may use just one of the support strategies outlined in this chapter or a combination of two, three, or 20 strategies. It may be hard work, but supporting your plan is *absolutely essential to its success.*

In Step 7—the final step in this method—you are asked to consider a few ideas and techniques that may help you on your journey. The intent here is to put your plan into action and then keep the momentum going.

So how do you keep yourself on track and support your plan?

Any process that works for you, either the one suggested in this book or a plan found elsewhere, is a good process—the important thing is to construct a support system that will keep you focused on your goals and will welcome optimal health, enduring happiness, peaceful prosperity, and thus a constructive evolution.

Following are some strategies, techniques, and suggestions, broken down into the Inner and Outer Realms, for supporting your HeLP and ensuring your success.

Don't feel that you have to use all of these strategies—just pick the ones that speak to you now, and save the others for a rainy day!

Use the chart at the end of this chapter to organize the strategies you choose for each goal you identified in Step 6.

Support Strategies 1: The Inner Realm

The strategies in this first section deal with your Inner Realm—that is, the inner workings of your mind. Use these strategies to consciously choose constructive mental intentions that support your HeLP.

Take a Leap of Faith

As part of your HeLP, you may have listed "calculated risk" as an ideal to welcome in. If you have done your prep work, become aware of various realities, and taken steps to forgive yourself and others, then you have put on the metaphoric helmet that will help protect you if you fall. If you haven't yet done so, then jump in! Take a leap of faith and enjoy the journey!

Re-declare Your Dedication to Change

Take a moment right now to review the Personal Declaration you filled out on page 11. Re-declare your dedication to working hard and doing whatever it takes to keep on welcoming a life of HHP. Review your compelling reason to change to remind yourself why you are dedicating your time and hard effort to this process.

Acknowledge Your Current Perfection

Accept yourself and acknowledge that you are perfect as you are. In your perfection, you are releasing certain habits and welcoming others. No matter where you are in your Unhealthyolic state, there is no place to go but up—that is, if you choose this path and work hard at it. Just remember the inspirational story of the cyclist Lance Armstrong, who was handed a death sentence. Despite the cancer raging through his body, Lance decided he was going to get better. And, boy, did he ever—he went on to win seven consecutive, grueling Tours de France. Wherever you start is the right place. You are great as you are, or at least you have greatness in you. Use whatever is *not* working in your life as a clue to help you decide what to welcome into your life. Your story going forward will be an inspiration to others.

Don't Resist

Besides accepting yourself in your current perfection, you must also take care not to resist whatever is going on in your life. Byron Katie (who, through a life-changing experience at the age of 44, developed a method of self-inquiry called "The Work") suggests that we do not resist what is and that we even "love what is."[33] For example, a person who is experiencing war either near or far should love what is happening. As radical as that sounds, that doesn't mean he should love war; it simply means he should be in a state of love and peace rather than of hate so that the war does not take over his mind. From that mindset, the person can then take action, like welcoming in a peaceful resolution. On a "lighter" note, if you have an Unhealthyolic habit of eating a box of doughnuts every day, then you must start by loving that that's the way it is—and from that point you can start welcoming HHP into your life.

Evaluate Your Current Values

In a nutshell, your values are the thoughts at the core of your thinking, the ones that matter most to you and take priority in your daily decisions.

These core values are a product of your inner mental programming and are like little mini-bosses that dictate what actions you take, who you hang out with, where you work, how you raise your children, and, especially, *how you affect your health, happiness, and prosperity.* You could spend lots of time trying to understand the values that currently rule your life. Perhaps you value what your parents taught you about lifestyle, or you value the system of

> ### Three Different Beliefs – The Same Value
>
> *Values are different from beliefs. Many people may value having good health but have different beliefs on how to be healthy.*
>
> *Nutritionally, omnivores believe humans are designed to eat a wide range of foods, including meat; a vegetarian believes in eating mostly cooked and raw vegetables, grains and fruits, and some animal products, such as eggs; a raw vegan believes that eating uncooked foods without a face is the best way to good health. All three have the same value of being healthy, but three different beliefs about how to get there.*

belief that was given to you by your culture or religion. Perhaps part of the reason you are an Unhealthyolic is that you *accepted without question* the guidance of your parents and elders or of institutions and "professionals."

If you live in alignment with your personal core values, you'll probably feel "happy" in your daily life, regardless of whether your values take on a positive or negative slant. For example, if one of your core values is "be kind to others" (positive), then you'd be likely to return a piece of lost jewelry you find. If your core value is "finders keepers" (negative), you may decide to keep the piece of jewelry. Either way, you'll feel good about your actions because they are in line with your core values.

Understanding what values you currently live by may explain your current life conditions. Your values will tell you why you've had the Unhealthyolic habits you've had until this point in your life. Even if you feel good about a negative value, you need to take a good, hard look at your values and determine whether or not your value system is working for you.

Ask yourself a few important questions:

- Am I okay with my current state of HHP?

- Do I feel happy most of the time?

- Is my body as healthy as it can be, with few, if any, sick days?

- Is my mind regularly crystal clear?

- Am I emotionally stable?

- Do I have a prosperous, low-stress life?

- Do I have a sense of purpose?

- If my answer to any of the above is no, do I have a plan to help my current state?

- Will my values support my plan?

If you answered no to any of these questions, then your current system may contain too many destructive values. You need to ask yourself if any of your values are causing a lack of health, happiness, and prosperity.

Let's look at some examples of possible destructive values and the consequences they may have in your life.

Value: I value financial success at all costs.
Consequence: You may have great riches but poor health, lousy relationships, and/or a deep bitterness.

Value: I value winning at all costs.
Consequence: You "win" at the cost of harming self, others, or the earth. Consider what winning means to you. Does it mean beating someone else or does it mean beating your own most recent "life score"? Suppose you have two athletes of equal attributes: the one whose only goal is to defeat the competition won't have as much power as the one trying to beat the world record to demonstrate the best potential of the current world population.

Value: Hanging out with my friends is a priority for me.
Consequence: You have a great relationship with your buddies, but your family wonders where you are every night. The situation causes many problems at home, which makes you feel uneasy.

Value: It's essential to me to belong to a certain group.
Consequence: You are part of an alliance that shares your values, beliefs, theologies, and ideologies, but it also has an isolated position in society; from this position you witness a world at war with every other "my-way-is-the-only-way" alliance.

Value: I value eating what I want, as much as I want, when I want.
Consequence: Your eating habits cause weight issues and other health problems.

If reading these examples has led you to realize that perhaps your values *are not* working for you, that's okay. You are allowed to change your values, to tear them down and build new ones. You are both a left-brain critical thinker and a right-brain intuitive being. Both your logic and your gut tell you that it's time to change, time to evolve.

Do not dwell on any of your "destructive" values; throw them into the shredder, forgive, gain wisdom, and move on. After all, if you trip on something while walking on a path, it's more important to look forward to see where to plant your next step securely than to look back at what you tripped on. It's behind you now!

Instead, ask yourself what values you strive for and be clear about which values inspire you and support you to move forward. Since you've already done your HeLP (haven't you?), you already have values seeded into you that will welcome a life of good health, happiness, and prosperity.

Remember that values are the thoughts at the core of your thinking, the ones that matter most to you and take priority in your daily decisions. Use your HeLP to guide new values. For example, the first "value" in the Relationship section of your HeLP may read, "I value loving myself. I value keeping the relationship with myself strong. I value being easy on myself. I value forgiving myself for any harm done to others by me or done to me." For a constructive life, turn the ideas in your HeLP into the new little mini-bosses that will support you.

Be Present

Even though Being Present may be in your HeLP, it's a helpful reminder that being aware of and living in the present moment is a key to HHP. You've heard it before: it's not the destination that matters, it's the journey. Eckhart Tolle captures this essence beautifully in his book *A New Earth:* "When you are Present, when your attention is fully in the Now, that Presence will flow into and transform what you do. There will be quality and power in it."[34]

Tapping into the present moment is like tapping into atomic energy. If you are tempted to give in to destructive habits that you chose to control, take a moment to focus on your breathing or your heartbeat, or both. This will help you control the temptation of your destructive instincts and mischievous IMP.

Believe

When two people of equal caliber start off from an equal place, the one who believes in herself will have the better chance of reaching the designated goal. Create belief. Fill your brain with thoughts that will help you believe in your vision and give you a reason to move forward.

Always Ask the Simple Question

By now you know that the most important question a HealthyIst can ask is a simple one: *Is this thought or action ultimately helping me, others, and/ or the earth toward a calm and kind, healthy, happy, and prosperous evolution (or is it at least neutral)?* If the answer is no, recognize and release the unhelpful thought and replace it with constructive thoughts and actions. If you cannot be directly constructive then support someone or an institution that can. For example, if you cannot grow your own food, instead of buying food that is shipped thousands of miles to put on your dinner plate, support vendors at a farmer's market that sell local produce and prepared foods.

> **Make the HealthyIsm Life Plan YOUR Plan!**
>
> You **do not** have to agree with every statement or idea listed, but **do** consider each one. The ideas in this book are my personal HealthyIsm Life Plan goals that I welcome as my values; as I move forward I do my best to use each one to help me evolve as a human being. If some ideas come across as too idealistic or unrealistic for you, then just focus on the ones that make sense to you.

Practice a State of Calmness

Even in the most chaotic moment, being in a state of calmness will make the journey so much better. Be calm on your quest for optimal health. As a martial artist, I know that the calmer you are in a confrontation, the better your chances of controlling the situation. If you have a lousy day that does not go as you planned, at least try to be calm. In your calmness you will have a better chance for clarity and for recognizing the next step.

Practice Perpetual Forgiveness and Unconditional Love

When we offer perpetual forgiveness, what we find on the other side of that coin is unconditional love. Perpetual forgiveness means automatically forgiving all transgressions forever. Having and giving unconditional love puts us in a higher state of consciousness of happiness and serenity. As humans, this is ultimately what we are looking for in most of our Unhealthyolic behaviors. Always start with yourself: look yourself in the eyes and offer unconditional love regardless of your own witness to your regretful thoughts, actions, and habits.

Practice Positive Affirmations

Developing a positive mindset is one of the most powerful life strategies there is. Positive affirmations promote constructive thinking.

When you read through the HeLP that you've developed, you are affirming a positive and constructive mindset. Use the HeLP Key Points Chart at the end of this chapter to remind you of the four basic affirmations:

- I am calmly aware.

- I am well in body, mind, and soul.

- I nurture my relationships.

- I build and maintain my resources.

More on Affirmations

You may not know it, but you have already developed a set of affirmations. Every thought you think and every word you say is an affirmation. Your "self-talk," or inner dialogue, is a stream of affirmations. We are all continually affirming subconsciously with our words and thoughts, and this flow of affirmations is what formulates our values and creates our life experience in every moment. Our values and beliefs are just learned thought patterns that we have been developing and affirming since childhood. Many of them work well for us, but others may now be dysfunctional and working against us, perhaps even sabotaging our efforts to achieve HHP.

Everything we think or say is a reflection of our inner truth or beliefs. It is important to realize that many of these "inner truths" may not actually be true for us now or may be based on invalid or inappropriate impressions we constructed as children, which if examined as an adult can be exposed as inappropriate.

Welcome making your self-talk loving and helpful toward HHP rather than destructive. Since many of your subconscious affirmations may be negative, the trick is to focus on the positive ones and to develop more of them. To do so, you can use "positive affirmations," which are short, positive statements that target a specific subconscious set of beliefs. Their purpose is to challenge and undermine negative beliefs and to replace them with positive, self-nurturing beliefs.

Remember that your HeLP is in an affirmation format in which each statement is a kind of "positive brainwashing"—that is, the affirmations help wash the negative beliefs away.

Visualize

Imagine that you are healthy, happy, and prosperous. At various points throughout the day, stop and take a moment to see yourself already "there." Visualize feeling energized, strong, glowing with good health, creating abundance in your life, sleeping well, breathing deeply and easily, eating great, and having a permanent smile on your face.

Think Critically

Thinking critically means using a mix of scientific evidence, gut feeling, and common sense to make decisions and take actions.

At your core, you may have values that are destructive; however, as we mature beyond the influential and immature years of childhood, we are able to think critically and use willpower to "do the healthy thing," which is to overcome unhealthy habitual values and develop empowering ones. Humanity itself is also maturing and beginning to make informed and intuitive choices based on what is best for all. Individually and as a whole, we are growing up.

Take 100% Responsibility

Perhaps up until this point you have allowed others to be responsible for your HHP—but from this point forward, you are in control! It's so easy for us to blame others for the hardships and handicaps we face. But for every story of a person who had a horrible upbringing or currently lives with a terrible situation, there is a story of someone who has prevailed in even worse circumstances. I am not belittling what you are going through; I am only asking you to fuel your path forward with the power of being the captain of your vessel—and that is the power of being 100% responsible. Commit to making it work.

Depend on Yourself

That's right—you are your own best support system. While it is wonderful and complimentary to have the support of your loved ones and others, you are the only person who completely understands and cares deeply about your goals. As you begin your journey, refer often to the work you did in the first six steps and use this book to keep you focused.

Never Say Never

If your IMP is screaming at you about the horrors of quitting your Unhealthyolic behaviors, then perhaps this approach may help. Tell yourself (your IMP) that every once in a while you will treat yourself to your indulgence, whether it be a favorite unhealthy food, a favorite mind-numbing television show, or being lazy for more than your allotted "lazy time." If this occasional indulgence has little or no consequence, then go ahead and tell yourself that you will allow that unhealthy behavior once a week, once a month, or once a year. But if you find yourself hooked again and unable to stop the unhealthy behavior after that supposed one-time indulgence—or if the Unhealthyolic behavior is something like taking hard drugs or gambling that will have serious HHP consequences—then tell your IMP that it may have a treat…in 50 years.

Keep Climbing the Mountain of HHP

Yes, it may be a big mountain, and it may take hard work, but your brain will adapt to your new pattern of behavior. For example, if you find that eating healthy is difficult for the first few days, you'll see that your brain will be well adapted to such a diet by the ninetieth day. Keep your eyes on the summit and on the goals you're aiming for. And know as you climb that your body is getting stronger and more energized, and that the mental view keeps getting better and better. Do not stop until you get to the top!

Learn to Say *No*

Whenever you find your IMP smooth-talking you into indulging in an unhealthy habit, become aware of the chatter, be strong, and just say no. No is a powerful word that will stop the craving, at least momentarily. Tell yourself that if you indulge, you may have a moment of pleasure, but memory reminds you that you won't feel good afterward. There are many stories of heroin addicts who successfully overcome their dependence on the highly addictive drug by learning to say no, digging in their heels, and never giving in to their physical cravings or their screaming IMP.

Control Your IMP Through the Aware Hand (AH) Method

As we saw in the previous chapters, one of the major keys to making your new lifestyle work for you is to gain control over your IMPish mind. You need to learn how to use your mind, rather than simply letting your mind use you. By being more involved with your thoughts and actions, and directing your mind to where you want and need it to go, you will be able to evolve your mind, body, and spirit—and your entire life—into the next stage of human development, which is to live in a constructive, healthy, happy, and prosperous existence.

To start, we are going to take the focus away from unhealthy lifestyle practices and their consequences and direct it toward the Aware Hand (AH) Method of controlling those unhealthy tendencies. This method can be used any time you find yourself falling into a destructive instinct or a programmed action or thought such as:

- Retaliating against a person who cuts you off in traffic

- Yelling back at someone who is provoking you

- Eating a tub of ice cream as a way of dealing with unpleasant emotion

- Judging someone because of his or her position in life, be it rich or poor, black or white, Jewish or Muslim

- Wanting to smoke a joint because something (like coming across a pack of matches in your junk drawer) triggered the craving

- Automatically sitting on your coach and flicking on the TV because that's what you've always done as an escape from your weight problems or other responsibilities

- Running out to the mall to buy something, even when you are in deep debt, as the result of some emotional trigger

Even the most "awake" person who knows he is in "control" of his IMP can falter at times and experience moments of being only partially aware. It is in those precise moments that he is in danger of sliding back into preprogrammed thoughts and actions. The AH Method, however, offers a visual and physical way to take back control of the IMP, stay on track, and transfer the negative energy into positive energy.

The method centers around the hands, which have long been considered a symbol of healing power (as in reiki) and as instruments of healing (as used by physiotherapists, massage therapists, and shiatsu practitioners). In his book *Anatomy of the Soul,* Rabbi Chaim Kramer also notes the special powers of the hands, and a symbol in Jainism shows a hand with a wheel on the palm that represents, among other things, the relentless pursuit of truth.[35] The AH Method also represents this pursuit but more in terms of the in-the-moment awareness of your thoughts and instincts, and the truth about the consequences of holding on to them.

The method consists of using the palm of one hand to expose any destructive IMP and its Unhealthyolic "chatter-energy" of the moment, and then to absorb it. You imagine that the chatter evolves into a constructive, loving, useful energy as your palm absorbs it. Then you focus on your heart. By placing your other hand on your heart, you transfer the new, evolved power into your heart. You then use this supportive power to ask yourself, "What is the one thought or action that I can do right now that will best serve me or others?"

The detailed steps below will guide you in your first experience with the AH Method.

Steps for Using the AH Method

Follow these steps whenever you catch yourself doing or thinking something that you now know does not serve you and which you no longer want to do.

1. Look at your hands and focus specifically on your *palms*.

2. Declare the palms of your hands an *instrument of awareness*—not just your personal awareness but also the awareness of Universal Spirit/God.

3. Point one of your palms toward your head. This action represents "pointing to the stream of thought" to show observance and awareness of your thoughts. You can raise your hand close to your head or leave it in an inconspicuous spot.

4. Envision your palm actually monitoring the unwelcome thought and action. Smile at the programmed action or thought and ask yourself, "Is this thought or action ultimately helping the optimal evolution of myself, others, and/or the world?"

5. Sit with the thought for a moment and just experience the feelings, desires, and emotions it brings up. Recognize the power of the picture that the programmed thought is painting in your head. For example, you may think, "If I drink that bottle of wine, I will be smiling and happy," or "If I cut that guy off who just cut me off, I will be the 'winner'."

6. As you continue to point your palm toward your head, say to the programmed thought, your IMP, "I see you, I am aware of your game," and then, "Thank you, but no thank you; you do not serve me."

7. Then imagine capturing the energy of that destructive thought in your hand. Place your hand on your chest and transfer the energy into your heart.

8. Now focus on your heartbeat and feel the power of your pulse.

9. Finally, "plant" a serving thought in your mind, such as, "What is the one thought or action I can do right now that will best serve me or others?"

Sally's Sample Scenario

1. Sally finds herself thinking about buying a tub of ice cream as a "treat" for completing a stressful day at work.

2. Sally knows that the ice cream isn't really just a treat, because she'd been abusing her body with too much ice cream and other junk food ever since she broke up with her cheating boyfriend. Her cat had died around the same time, leaving her completely alone.

3. Over time, Sally has become aware of her destructive thinking and is now using the AH Method to catch and control non-serving thoughts.

4. She points her palm toward her head to represent her

awareness of the thought.

5. She sits with the thought for a while and recognizes the resulting feelings that it brings.

6. She then says to the thought, "I see you, I am aware of your game," and then, "Thank you, but no thank you; you do not serve me."

7. She then envisions grabbing the energy of the non-serving thought with her hand. She places her hand on her chest and transfers the energy to her heart.

8. After a moment, Sally takes a deep breath and counts the heartbeats in the breath cycle. She feels more relaxed.

9. She then asks herself, "What is the one thought or action that I can do right now that will best serve me or others?"

10. With new energy, a sudden thought pops into her head: "I'll go for a brisk, energizing walk."

Once you become accustomed to using the AH Method, you'll find that you no longer need to perform the actual physical movement of the palms pointing toward the head; instead, you can just envision it. Eventually you will simply be aware of all the IMP thoughts in your mind and find yourself answering the ultimate question even before you ask it.

I Forgive

"To err is human; to forgive, divine."

This quote by Alexander Pope demonstrates that we humans make mistakes and the best way to move on is to forgive self and others. The avatars of the past knew it, Pope knew it, and it's time for all of us to know it now: forgiving self and others is a key to our own optimal HHP and that of the rest of the earth. The moment you truly forgive is a moment of relief and peace for you. Practice saying the words in your own language: "I forgive you. I forgive me. I forgive whoever or whatever!" At the end of each day, before going to sleep, say to all the people on earth, "I forgive you," for whatever wrongs they have done. No person was born with the intent to do wrong. It's only through destructive instincts and IMP that they "progress" to that point.

Learn to say "I forgive" in different languages as well, especially if you belong to a nation or religion or community that holds a grudge against another. A few examples:

> French: je pardonne
> Spanish: yo perdono
> Italian: io perdono
> Japanese: watash yurushimasu
> German: ich verzeihe

American Sign Language: with the tips of the fingers of one hand, make two light strokes along the length of the other hand from palm to fingers.

Support Strategies 2: The Outer Realm

The strategies in this section deal with your Outer Realm—that is, the place where your physical actions influence your environment. Use these strategies to consciously manifest the actions that will support your HeLP.

Shut Off or Filter *All* Media

To support aiming for your HeLP, you must control what images filter into your brain. If you repeatedly see or hear of someone else's belief, it may become yours, too. For example, if you watch a certain news channel that is owned by a corporation that is also in the business of selling specific products, services, or beliefs, it may present to you a reality that is favorable to its agenda. Be careful of what streams into your conscious and unconscious mind.

Gather Knowledge

You have likely heard the expression "knowledge is power," which usually means that the more knowledge or education you have, the more potential you will have in life. This concept extends to your HHP as well. The more you know about what it takes to be healthy, what truly makes you happy, and how to be prosperous, the better your potential for HHP.

Be aggressive and gather as much information as you can handle, then make decisions based on all the information. You can also use this book as a guide and starting point, but don't rely on it; make sure you do your own research and critical thinking.

Explore Motivational Material

Read or listen to materials that motivate you toward controlling your Unhealthyolic habits, and keep the energy going as you aim for HHP. Use a variety of materials like books, DVDs, MP3 downloads, CDs, and newsletters—or just choose one that works best for you. (For a list of recommended motivational materials, go to HealthyIsm.com.)

Be Your Own Best Nutritionist, Fitness Trainer, and Health Expert

Save the professionals for when you really need them. As you move through life, get to know what works best for you in terms of nutrition and exercise. Also get to know the health of your body and learn to understand when it offers signs or symptoms of a deficiency or toxicity.

Use a Key Points Chart to Keep You Focused on the HeLP

We tend to get lost in our busy thoughts and day-to-day challenges, which can cause confusion and make us lose sight of what it is we're welcoming into our lives. To help keep your attention focused and intentions clear, use the work you did on your HealthyIsm Life Plan to develop a Key Points Chart.

On a sheet of paper or on your computer, record in short form what thoughts and actions you are welcoming on a daily basis. This chart should include the four affirmations from Step 6, the main goals you listed on your HeLP, and the strategies you chose to reach those goals. Be sure to include your compelling reason to change, too! Be brief in your summary—the purpose of the chart is only to refresh your memory and to use as a point of focus.

Each morning, before you look at your HeLP, remind yourself of your compelling reason to change. Then look at your Key Points Chart and declare: *This is who I am and who I will happily maintain or welcome today.* At the end of the day, ask yourself if you gave 100% (or less) of your best energy to maintaining or welcoming. It doesn't matter if you did or didn't give 100%; if you didn't reach your goal, just forgive yourself. Start fresh every day. Keep practicing.

Now all you have to do is place a copy of your Key Points Chart in lots of different places. Put one by your bed, desk, and bathroom mirror, as well as in your car and in your wallet—whatever you have to do to keep your HealthyIsm Life Plan foremost in your mind. (See the end of this chapter for a sample Key Points Chart.)

Reward Yourself as You Improve

Acknowledge and reward yourself for each Unhealthyolic habit you overcome. Perhaps you can put a little money aside every time you achieve a goal (or a portion of a goal) on your HeLP, and then treat yourself to a vacation, a massage, a maid service, or a healthy restaurant meal. At least pat yourself on the back!

Immunize Yourself Against Negative People and Dogmas

Create a shield that will not let the negativity of others' thoughts and actions get to you. You may find that as you overcome your Unhealthyolic habits, other people may be somewhat uncomfortable with you; their reaction is simply a combination of their primal survival mode and their IMP fearing that they'll be controlled next.

Look at chaos from others as a "negativity virus vaccine." Treat all the negativity, failures, challenges, and pessimism of others as booster shots to your willpower that will continue to make you stronger until you completely immunize yourself against the "negativity virus." Create a negativity immune system to keep the "virus" out.

Surround Yourself with Constructive People

Hang out with people *who support your HHP habits,* who talk the HHP talk, and who walk the HHP walk. When you live unconsciously (when your IMP and instincts are in control), you usually hang out with people who support your Unhealthyolic habits—but to succeed, you must change that! If you have no one around you who can support your new HHP habits, or you are looking for an extra boost, join up with supportive people on HealthyIsm.com.

Do Physical Exercise

When you feel the urge to indulge in an Unhealthyolic behavior, get up and get moving. Go for a walk, a bike ride, a run, a swim, climb a hill, climb a tree (be careful!), lift weights, plant a garden, build something with wood, or do anything else that gets your blood flowing. Using your body will send natural endorphins into your bloodstream that will give you a euphoric feeling and may alleviate the craving. Use physical exercise to create a HealthyIsm Retreat, as described next.

Create a HealthyIsm Retreat in Your Home

Take a look around your home and remove the temptations—unhealthy foods, drugs, alcohol, unlimited television viewing—that fed the Unhealthyolic habits that you are in the process of controlling. Replace them with things that will help you, like supportive literature, vibrant food, exercise equipment, and selective (or no) television viewing. (See HealthyIsm.com for help with building a retreat in your home.)

Team Up With a Coach or a Coaching Group

Just as an athletic coach supports and enhances sporting skills, a life coach helps pull the best out of you. Having a personal life coach gives you a sounding board and accountability partner, someone who can offer you a wide range of experience, tools, and resources to help you make a smooth transition to a constructive lifestyle. If you can't find a suitable coach in your area, then team up with a HealthyIsm Life Coach through the HealthyIsm.com website.

Register for a HealthyIsm Retreat

If you need a boot camp that will kick you into high gear as you aim for the goals set out in your HeLP, register for one of the HealthyIsm Retreats offered through the HealthyIsm website. Programs are available for three days, one week, or the recommended 21 days. During your retreat, you will continue to refine your HeLP, learn to eat well, learn to exercise properly, and reconnect with your original nature-self. A recommended prerequisite is to have read through the *HealthyIsm* book at least once. (For more information, see the HealthyIsm Retreat page on HealthyIsm.com.)

Connect With Others on the HealthyIsm Website

The HealthyIsm website is a great place to connect with a community of people who are on the same path as you toward finding supporting thoughts, actions, habits, and goals that kindly and calmly help themselves, others, or the earth toward an HHP evolution. Tune in to others on the same quest through videos, webinars, and forums. Most of the resources are offered free of charge, but you are asked to pass on what you have learned—and the freedom from Unhealthyolic habits that you've gained—to at least two other people.

A Few More Things

As you continue your journey to a life of HealthyIsm, keep the following in mind.

Practice + Persistence + Time = Stronger Willpower = Success

Just like working the muscles of your body makes them stronger, using your willpower will make it stronger over time. Michael Jordan, who didn't make his high school basketball team, dedicated tons of time, practiced continuously, and stayed persistent—and then he went on to have one of the world's most successful sports careers of all time. If you practice your plan and persist over time, you and your goals will gain even more support.

Be Open to Change or Improve Your Plan

If you find something that makes better rational and intuitive sense and will help you overcome your Unhealthyolic habits more easily, then make the change. Look continuously for ways to improve your HeLP, and let it grow with you.

Do What Works Best for You

Try making changes cold turkey at first. If that doesn't work, then go more slowly and work your way into the changes. Use whatever method works best for you. Most importantly, embrace the new energy when it comes your way—and know that it will come! You may be plugging away at HHP and feel concerned because you don't see or feel any difference—and then one day, all of a sudden, you feel amazing, your thinking is clear, abundance is flowing, and your pains go away. Smile, embrace it, and move faster toward an optimal lifestyle. But be careful—your IMP may say to you, "You are doing so well; have a treat!"

Our lives are a co-creation of our choices and our interaction with acts of nature/Universal Spirit/God and with the choices and actions of others.

It's time to control our choices and for in-your-face tough love with ourselves—not with our children, our neighbors, or other nations! If we want to make our new, constructive lifestyles work, then we have to work on the *I*.

The next chapter will be a review of the work you have done to this point—or perhaps you've been skimming through the book looking for a quick fix. Either way, you'll discover that controlling your choices in life might be as easy as brushing your teeth.

Shayne's Story of Persistence
"We are all just differently capable"

*When Shayne was 4 months old he was struck with a bacterial infection that rapidly destroyed parts of his body and was given a 2% chance of surviving. With the never give up attitude of his mother, a team of medical doctors, and Shayne's persistence, he not only survived the deadly challenge but today leads a rewarding life. Even though he lost both legs around the knee, part of one arm, tips of his remaining hand and other pieces of his body he is a respected top player on Canada's wheelchair basketball team shooting 80% from the three point line. Whether training for the 2012 Paralympics, helping kids with their own **challenges** or giving high energy, motivational talks to corporations, he always repeats his mantra – "we are **all** just differently capable".*

*If you ever think that you just can't do it, remember this inspiring man and continue with your quest for a constructive life. For more information on Shayne, or to have him motivate your **differently capable** group to score from the **three point line** of their challenges, visit HealthyIsm.com.*

HealthyIsm: *Healthy I, Healthy World!*

Step 7 Exercise: Support Strategies for Your HeLP

List your goals from the GOAL column of the Step 6 HeLP that you created. Next to each, write in at least one SUPPORT STRATEGY you'll use to help keep yourself on track and ensure success for that goal. Try to use both Inner and Outer Realm strategies. You might repeat the same strategy for more than one goal. An example has been provided.

HeLP GOAL from Step 6	SUPPORT STRATEGY: Inner Realm	SUPPORT STRATEGY: Outer Realm
I physically use my body in many ways.	*Visualize: I visualize my healthy-looking and healthy-feeling body. I take 100% responsibility for it.*	*I explore motivational material. I will listen to materials that will motivate me to get off my butt and get moving.*

HeLP Key Points Chart (Sample)

This sample chart is based on the HeLP developmental work you completed in Steps 1–6. Use this as a guide as you create your own Key Points Chart. A blank chart has been provided on the next page. See bottom of page 223 for more information.

Compelling Reason to Change

Example: My compelling reason to change is that I have had enough of living a mediocre life, and I am tired of the destruction in the world. I want to calmly and kindly welcome optimal health, enduring happiness, and peaceful prosperity for self and for the world.

AFFIRMATION 1: I Am Calmly Aware			
Present moment	Hidden agendas	IMP's control	Mental chemistry
Physical chemistry	Physical messages	In tune with food	Higher source
General evolutionary purpose	Specific personal purpose	Direction	Death not to be feared
Destructive instincts	Rhythm of my body and the environment	Silver linings	Global shift in consciousness

AFFIRMATION 2: I Am Well in Body, Mind, and Soul			
Multi-functional exercise	Just enough exercise	Proper fuel	Just enough fuel
Enough sunshine	Toxin-free	Treat control	Mental-robics
Positive mental support	Meditate, pray, or focus often	Sleepy time	Quiet rest
Laugh, dance, sing, and play	Emotional health		

HealthyIsm: *Healthy I, Healthy World!*

AFFIRMATION 3: I Nuture My Relationships			
Love myself	My "true" love	Love my coworker	Love my family
Love earth	Love Universal Spirit or God	Love my neighbor, community, world	Charity partnership

AFFIRMATION 4: I Build and Maintain Resources			
My thoughts	Good questions	Communication	Good health
Intuition	Support network	Wisdom	Talents
Jolly job	Productivity	Cash and assets	Getaway places
Tools for daily life	Willpower	Forgiveness	Less clutter
The Internet	Stress	Stress releasers	Truth
Self-defense	Sacrifice	Time	Earth
Peace	Calculated risk	Choice	My HeLP

My HeLP Key Points Chart

Compelling Reason to Change

_____
_____
_____
_____

AFFIRMATION 1: I Am Calmly Aware			

AFFIRMATION 2: I Am Well in Body, Mind, and Soul			

HealthyIsm: *Healthy I, Healthy World!*

AFFIRMATION 3: I Nurture My Relationships			

AFFIRMATION 4: I Build and Maintain Resources			

Quick Fix!

There is nothing so easy but that it becomes difficult when you do it reluctantly.
—Terence, Roman comic dramatist

*There's no easy way out.
If there were, I would have bought it.
And believe me, it would be one of my favorite things!*
—Oprah Winfrey

Most people are about as Healthy, Happy, and Prosperous as they make up their minds to be.

—Borrowed from Abraham Lincoln:
*Most folks are about as happy
as they make up their minds to be.*

Note: Readers who have read the book to this point may wish to use this chapter as a review.

HealthyIsm: *Healthy I, Healthy World!*

So you read through the table of contents and the words "Quick Fix" just jumped out at you. And now here you are—or should I say, here is where your inner mental programming (IMP) brought you. In that case...

Hello, IMP—good to see you! I understand that you are looking for a quick fix for stopping your Unhealthyolic habits and welcoming health, happiness, and prosperity (HHP) into your life—something fast, so you don't have to waste your time.

Well, then, without further ado, here is the three-step, quick-fix plan:

Step 1
Ask yourself the simple question: *Are my thoughts, actions, habits, or goals neutral or ultimately helping me, others, and/or the earth to welcome a calm and kind, healthy, happy, and prosperous evolution?*

Step 2
If your answer is yes: Quick fix accomplished! Congratulations! You're already a HealthyIst, so take a break, put this book down, and go do something good for yourself, others, or the planet!

Step 3
If your answer is *no*: You will need to dedicate yourself and your willpower to transforming your destructive thoughts and actions into constructive forces. If you're not sure how to do that, then *go back to Chapter 1 and get started on your road to HealthyIsm!*

CHAPTER 12. *QUICK FIX!*

As you might have guessed by the tongue-in-cheek three-step plan above, there is no "quick fix" for an unhealthy lifestyle and destructive habits. Truly committing to a life of HealthyIsm takes time, passion, determination, and perseverance. Most of us learn at some point in our lives that supposed "shortcuts" to health, wealth, and happiness—the ubiquitous get-rich-quick schemes and miracle diets—rarely work and often result in the exact opposite of the desired outcome.

That said, you may still think that you simply don't have the time to go through the exercises presented in the seven steps in this book. Perhaps you want to bypass the preliminaries and go directly for the gusto. For you, the quick fix may be a potential—but temporary—solution.

This chapter was originally written to ask the question, *Is there a quick way to "fix" Unhealthyolic behaviors and quickly achieve an HHP life?* And the short answer to that question is *no*. Although many promotional strategies in the quick-fix, self-improvement marketplace may appeal to our lazy natures and tempt us to buy products that promise immediate gratification, the truth is that there is no pill, self-help book, DVD, course, or seminar that produces the same results as determined *effort*. Just as it takes hard work and exercise to properly build muscle and shed unnecessary body fat, it takes focused effort and willpower to release destructive habits and welcome HealthyIsm into your life.

In fact, the quickest way to start living a constructive life *is to make a conscious shift in your mind,* right now, that no matter what, you will control your thoughts with steadfast determination and find a way to welcome HHP into your life.

If you have read the book to this point and have completed the exercises in each step, use the following as a review; if you haven't read the book, the summaries of each step below will give you the basic groundwork for beginning to transform your Unhealthyolic habits. However, I do encourage you to read the book in its entirety, because it may offer you many seeds of support that will help you on your quest.

If you are still determined to just "get to the crunch of it," then start by reading the summary of Step 1 and asking yourself, "Can I clearly and easily answer the questions?" If the answer is yes, move on to the next step, and so on. If you read a step you don't understand, go to the corresponding chapter and examine it.

Step 1: What Happened to Us?

In this step you look at destructive instincts and the beliefs, patterns, and experiences that contributed to your destructive behaviors. You are introduced to your IMP (inner mental programming), the grand-daddy of all the reasons we develop Unhealthyolic behaviors.

Answer the following questions:

- Are you aware of how your inner mental programming—the input from people and institutions, including all of your life experiences and lessons—controls your life today?

- Are you aware of destructive instincts that contribute to your Unhealthyolic habits today?

If you answered yes to both questions, and if you understand everything that happened to you and how it led you into a state of unhealthiness, unhappiness, and scarcity, then move on to Step 2. If you could not answer the questions, take a moment to read Chapter 5 and reflect on Step 1.

Step 2: What's Your Current Truth?

What is your truth? In this step you take a bird's-eye view of your life and look honestly at what is good and what is not. You discover what it means to have a calm awareness of the way you think and act, and consider whether or not you give your physical, mental, and spiritual bodies the right elements to develop and maintain them. You take a critical look at your relationship level with self, significant other, charities, family, other people, plants and animals, spirituality, and so on. And you assess the tools, resources, and assets you have to work with, such as good health, business sense, knowledge, talents, physical strength, languages, and global connectivity.

Answer the following questions:

- How aware are you of all aspects of your life today?

- Are you aware of the present moment, of the hidden agendas of others, and of your IMP?

- Are you aware of what you eat and how it affects your mind and body?

- Do you know the best way to keep your body, mind, and soul healthy?

- Do you have healthy relationships with yourself, Universal Spirit/God, and all others around you?

- Do you have resources to support an HHP life, such as a job you love, productivity, good health, a life blueprint, global connectivity through the Internet, a healthy amount of stress, and truth?

If you are clear on the *shape* of your life at this moment, then move on to Step 3; if not, then read Chapter 6 and follow the Step 2 exercises.

Step 3: Zoom Out—Review Your Overall Past

Step 2 is all about taking a bird's-eye view of your life as it is *today*. In Step 3, you look at your *past* from birth to the present. You consider your personal life and what has influenced or touched you physically, mentally, and spiritually, both positively and negatively. As you remember and record your past, you also record whatever comes up from your subconscious.

Answer the following questions:

- Which memories of your life experiences, upbringing, schooling, events, and so on—both good and bad, recent and long past—seem to have influenced or touched you most in your life?

- What have others done for you or to you—both for better and for worse—from your birth to your present life? What have you done to or for others and yourself?

If the answers to these questions are clear, move on to Step 4. If not, review Step 3 in Chapter 7.

Step 4: Zoom In—Reveal Your Messy Past

Welcoming an HHP life can be significantly easier when you know if there is anything in your past that causes you to act the way you do today. In Step 4 you "zoom in" on the messy, destructive, or otherwise negative memories from Step 3 and identify anything in your past that needs to be laid to rest so that it no longer affects your present life. (For example, if your father always said, "You're a klutz!" and you repeated that to yourself over the years, the hold that this memory has on you might need to be released.)

Answer the following questions:

- What are the key memories from Step 3 that may have a negative effect on your life today?

- Are there any dogmas or beliefs that you have today that were influenced by the thoughts and actions of others?

If you are fully aware of these messy areas, then go to Step 5 to find *R.E.L.I.E.F.* Otherwise, do the Step 4 exercises in Chapter 8.

Step 5: R.E.L.I.E.F.!

In Step 5, you take a list of destructive events, experiences, perceptions, teachings, actions, dealings, incidents, etc., from the past or present that may influence your life today, and you learn how to stop them from affecting your present life by following the step-by-step R.E.L.I.E.F. technique.

Answer the following questions:

- Do you have a method to release any mental manipulators of the past or present as they affect your life today?

- Are you able to forgive yourself and others and release past transgressions?

If you already have great HHP and feel no need for relief, then move on to Step 6. If you do need to release any manipulators in your life, go to Step 5 in Chapter 9 to practice the R.E.L.I.E.F. technique.

Step 6: Develop Your HealthyIsm Life Plan (HeLP)

In Step 6, imagine that you have just arrived on earth (at your current age and physical state and with whatever positive resources and relations you currently have), free of any emotional baggage and in full control of your IMP. You are in total control of your thinking and what you'd like to welcome into your life. From this point, you develop a plan to welcome HHP into your life. This HealthyIsm Life Plan (your HeLP) focuses on four key areas of your life: your awareness of various aspects of life; your body, mind, and soul; your relationships; and your resources.

Answer the following questions:

CHAPTER 12. *QUICK FIX!*

- Do you have a well-thought-out plan to welcome HHP into your life?

- Do you know what an HHP life looks like for you?

If you already have a life plan, go to the next step to lock it in and make it work. If you're unsure about your plan or don't know where to start, go back to Chapter 10 and complete the exercises in Step 6.

Step 7: Support Your HeLP

By the time you reach Step 7, you have released any control that mental manipulators have over your life and developed a HealthyIsm Life Plan to welcome HHP into your life. In Step 7, you "lock it in" and put on the finishing touches, so to speak. Just as an artist would finish her painting with a protective spray or a chef would top his beautiful food creation with a special sauce, you learn to support and protect your developed plan to encourage its fulfillment

Answer the following questions:

- Are you willing to do whatever it takes to welcome HHP into your life?

- Do you have a method or methods to welcome your detailed plan into your life?

If you are already supporting a well thought out life plan and you are doing whatever it takes to welcome HHP into your life then move on to the next Consideration. If you are not supporting your help go back to Chapter 11 and select as many techniques as possible to *help your HeLP.*

Regardless of where you are in the activity of life, welcoming and maintaining HHP is as easy as brushing your teeth. Through the evolution of the toothbrush to our loving parents showing us how to use it and coaxing us to do it thousands of times, we have learned to brush our teeth, like it or not. By now, it's not even a question of whether we will or we won't—we just do it. Think about it: it takes effort to buy a toothbrush and toothpaste, put yourself in front of the sink, pick up the toothbrush, rinse it, put toothpaste on it, raise it to your mouth, brush your teeth, rinse again, and so on—yet you do all of that unconsciously and almost effortlessly.

The point is that the quick fix to stopping your destructive habits and welcoming in optimal health, enduring happiness, and peaceful prosperity is as "easy" as brushing your teeth—that is, moving from need to thought to the development of a good habit, and then sticking to it.

All it takes is one thought to make this happen.

One thought…talk about a quick fix!

CONSIDERATION III

Receiving and Giving Support

As you practice HealthyIsm, you may find yourself either in need of support from others or in the honorable, magical, happy place of being able to support those who are still on their way to a constructive life or just beginning the process.

Whether you are on the giving or the receiving end of the support, both have the power to be constructive to the process of creating a healthy I and a healthy world. This Consideration addresses two of the most important aspects of HealthyIsm: the ability to receive with appreciation and the willingness to give with no expectations of receiving something in return (except the feeling of joy).

Welcoming In Support and Kindness

All of us, at certain moments of our lives, need to take advice and to receive help from other people.
—Alexis Carrel

Advice is seldom welcome, and those who need it the most, like it the least.
—Lord Chesterfield

My first thoughts are that I should not let people down, that I should support them and love them.
—Princess Diana

Bravo for making it this far! You've decided to be kind and supportive to yourself by taking control of your thoughts and your life! You are an evolutionary—developing and respecting your body and mind, assisting Mother Nature in her biological unfolding, welcoming in health, happiness, and prosperity (HHP).

Let's review what you have done up to now. You have become aware of various aspects of your life by identifying the happenings and experiences of the past and present that influence your thoughts and choices. You've become aware of your destructive instincts and challenged your inner mental programming (IMP), found R.E.L.I.E.F., and taken control of your IMP. You've created and welcomed into your life the components of a HealthyIsm Life Plan (HeLP), which produces an openness to receiving health, happiness, and prosperity. You are also doing everything possible to keep your HeLP on track.

If having completed the steps in this book has already enabled you to control your instincts and your thoughts and welcome HHP into your life, then for you these pages are just a preamble to the next chapter, "Giving Support and Kindness."

But what if your plan isn't working? What if it isn't helping you stop your Unhealthyolic habits and welcome in HHP? Perhaps you've found yourself feeling lonely, confused, and overwhelmed. Perhaps you're not sure if you're "doing it right" or you're in need of a little push. Perhaps you've been bombarded by negativity from others.

No matter which point you're at right now, it's time to consider possible ways of welcoming support and kindness from the world around you… sometimes *even when you would never expect it.*

Receiving the Giving

Of course, by reading and applying the concepts in this book, you have already begun to welcome in support and kindness. But the world is full of other sources of support and kindness that can help you stay on the right track and see you through tough times. This chapter lists just a few of the resources you'll find in the world around you. And note that you'll easily recognize a source of true support and kindness because it will be calmly and kindly helping you stop your Unhealthyolic habits and welcome improved HHP into your life.

Sun and Earth

One of the most basic ways of receiving the giving is to welcome in kindness and support from the sun and the ideal atmosphere of mother earth that supports life, which supports you.

All life on earth, from the wonderful human being to the breathtakingly immense variety of plants and animals, is supported by the nutrients and microbes of the soil and water below and the sun, air, and ideal temperature above. As in the "Dear Food" prayer in Chapter 10, acknowledge and welcome from Earth and sun any and all aspects that are kind and supportive to you.

Family

If a family member comes up to you and says something

like, "Wow, you are looking great," or "Good for you for kicking that habit—I am proud of you," or if they help you prepare a healthy meal or hold your hand or give you a hug in a hard moment, recognize the kindness and support, drink it in, and offer a simple response, such as "Thank you." If the person does not offer support and kindness but instead throws obstacles like pessimism, jealousy, or hatefulness into your path, you simply need to respond with an "Okay, I understand" and quietly accept them as they are within their own IMP and destructive instincts. Welcome in family kindness and support when offered to you, and acknowledge and learn from anything that is not intended to be constructive. Many people shrug off kindness and support with phrases like, "I can do it by myself," "I'm okay," or "I don't need your help." When you receive kindness and support, just say thank you and welcome it in. This is not to say that you should rely on or look forward to family members offering such compassion; it's just a reminder to welcome it in and accept it as it is.

Religion

If you are religious, welcome in any kindness and support from your religion that will help you practice a life of Healthy-Ism. But be conscious: some religions are based on an individual's or group's IMPish *interpretation* of life on this planet, the creator of that life, and what happens *after* life. Their interpretation is then re-interpreted by others. Welcome in the interpretations that do not cause destruction but that instead show control of one's instincts and IMP and that are about welcoming in HHP. If your religion can be interpreted in a peaceful, kind, supportive, and loving way to self and others...welcome it! If your religion causes you to have negative feelings and take destructive actions toward self or others, forgive the interpreter(s). Instead, develop your own calm and kind perception and interpretation that allows you to practice your religion *and* a life of Healthy-Ism—and to pass that on to the next person or generation.

Group Culture

Most of us grew up within a certain culture or mix of cultures. Cultures are rich in ancestral interpretations of *their* experiences of their reality in *their* part of the world during *their* time in history; how they developed values and practices, how they lived their lives, and how they prepared their children for life were all based on those interpretations. Some cultural practices are good; some are bad. Welcome in the good stuff; smile and forgive the rest. Be careful of holding onto cultural practices that are knowingly harmful, such as gender and race inequalities, early marriages, mutilations, and regularly and excessively eating certain culture foods that are known by modern nutritional sciences to damage the body. But do hold on to and welcome in the support and kindness of beneficial cultural practices such as language, dance, music and other artistic expressions, prolonged breast feeding, caring for the elderly and other members of the "village" in times of need, and so on.

Society

As we evolve as a society and learn as we go, we are developing certain methods and reasonable ways of living together. Welcome in support and kindness from the positive attributes that modern society offers, such as freedom, civility, cooperation, social stability, education, responsibility, and connection. Also welcome in any support to recover from weak states of mind or unhealthy bodies.

Society at one time may have had to fight over resources due to necessity, ignorance, or greed. But we have matured and are aware that, collectively and with cooperative global mind power, we can live together harmoniously and solve every imagined problem facing society. The mind power that we dedicate toward the fear of others and other IMP habits now has the opportunity to be channeled into stopping Unhealthyolic habits and welcoming in HHP.

If you are on the receiving end, use your mind power to welcome in whatever amount of support and kindness is given and continue practicing HealthyIsm.

But I usually do things for myself! It's hard for me to receive support and kindness!

Since the day you were born, you have been kindly supported in many ways by some or many people and things: by the life-giving force of Universal Spirit/God that created you; by the sun and its life-giving properties; by the earth and its provisions; by the fellowship and guidance of your religion, culture, and society; and by your family's love and nurturing.

And while it's true that some of this so-called support may have done you more harm than good, you are now at a new moment in your time on Earth. You are now aware of your destructive instincts and IMP and no longer allow negative experiences or the harmful agendas of others to affect you mentally or physically. You are now in a moment in which you will only welcome in constructive kindness and support.

To evaluate the types of kindness and support you are receiving in your new life of HealthyIsm, try the following exercise:

Exercise: Sources of Support and Kindness

- Take a quiet moment to close your eyes and be aware of the various kinds people, acts, and things that have constructively and positively supported and been kind to you up to now. Open your eyes and write down all of the sources you thought of.

- In addition to listing the precious resources of the Earth, sun, and beyond, include even the simple things that support you, such as the health of your immune system, the clothes you wear, the dwelling you live in, the bed you sleep in, your ability to communicate with others, and your body that supports you in a multitude of ways. You get the picture: open your senses and be aware of all the things that support your very existence.

- With this awareness, offer gratitude and the commitment that you won't receive gifts in vain. Also promise yourself and the world that you will endeavor to practice HealthyIsm at whatever pace you're capable of at this time.

Support from the HealthyIsm Organization

Besides happily contributing a considerable percentage of its profits toward helping others take control of their lives, the HealthyIsm Organization offers support and kindness in many other ways. It has a growing support community that consists of people who have already gone through the process, are in increasingly better control of their minds, and are fully welcoming in a life of HHP, or who are on the path to doing so. The HealthyIsm website contains helpful information, videos, and recordings that offer you support and kindness to welcome in HHP.

There are also links to pro-HealthyIsm professionals like medical doctors, naturopaths, chiropractors, wellness coaches, fitness trainers, and dieticians—and all of these professionals have worked on the *I* first and are welcoming HHP into their lives.

Below you will find information about the people, tools, services, and products that make up the HealthyIsm Organization and that you can turn to for kindness and support.

The HealthyIsm.com Website

This website is designed as an interactive focal point where people practicing HealthyIsm can find informative resources, guidance, and support for stopping their Unhealthyolic habits and welcoming in HHP. The website includes tools, services, and products such as the HealthyIsm book and fitness, nutrition, and meditation video and audio recordings.

Gary Drisdelle, author of HealthyIsm: Healthy I, Healthy World!

Gary is dedicated to giving kindness and support to others. He participates regularly in the forums, webinars, and newsletters, and also provides one-on-one support, keynote speeches, and seminars of various lengths. See the contact page at Healthy-

Ism.com for more information.

HealthyIsm Forums

The HealthyIsm forums are meeting places for people who have stopped or are in the process of stopping their Unhealthyolic habits and who are welcoming in HHP. Logging in at HealthyIsm.com provides access to the various forums.

Other Support and Kindness

Be sure to also seek out the growing number of people and organizations whose mission it is to offer support to others. Below is just a brief sampling of the other methods available that may offer you support and kindness on your journey to better control your life.

The Work by Byron Katie

As mentioned earlier in this book, Byron Katie has helped many people challenge their destructive thoughts and turn their lives around. Through a method of self-inquiry called The Work, a person is helped to *undo* thoughts that cause suffering.

Emotional Freedom Therapy

Developed by Gary Craig, Emotional Freedom Therapy (EFT) uses acupressure and suggestive affirmative talk as a method of releasing the hold your emotions may have on the health of your body and mind. The therapy is based on the same underlying thread of thought in this book: we are not our thoughts, and we are therefore not going to be dominated emotionally, mentally, or physically by our stubborn hold on disempowering thoughts.

The Philosophy of Eckhart Tolle

Tolle's latest book, *A New Earth,* reinforces the ideas presented in his original book, *The Power of Now,* which centers on the philosophy that most people are trapped in their self-created prison of thought. Tolle leads people out of this jail by helping them recognize the immense power of the moment through such exercises as awareness (not analysis) of their breath or the world around them.

More information and links to all of these materials and more are available at the HealthyIsm.com website.

Receiving *Is* Giving

To warmly allow someone to give to you is like giving a gift to them; it's like the completion of that person's good intentions. It gives them happiness. Think of a time when you wanted to give something to someone and he refused to receive it; it probably didn't feel very good. Recognize all the kindness and support available to you, move beyond pride, and welcome it in. Once you find yourself continuously welcoming HHP into your life, then go one step farther and be the giver, the creator of good intentions, and give back into the web and cycle of life by helping others stop their Unhealthyolic habits and welcome in HHP.

Giving Out Support and Kindness

If you can't feed a hundred people, then just feed one.
—Mother Teresa

*You get the best out of others when you
give the best of yourself.*
—Harvey S. Firestone

*To give without any reward, or any notice,
has a special quality of its own.*
—Anne Morrow Lindbergh

As humans mature, sooner or later we figure out that what goes around comes around. Most of us have heard that at the end of life it's not how much you acquired, it's how much you gave of yourself to others that you will remember and that others will remember of you. Giving selflessly of self is the most fulfilling, lasting, and pleasurable thing you can do; it's better than any drug, shopping spree, or favorite food.

Tikkun olam is a Hebrew saying that a kind neighbor of mine translated as "when you do good to something, you do good to everything, because everything is connected within the same web of life." I read elsewhere that *tikkun olam* also refers to the concept that people everywhere are not only responsible for helping their own, but also for helping others and *repairing the world*—that ultimately, all humans are responsible for each other.

Giving Support and Kindness

Because we are all interconnected in Mother Nature's web, by giving to others we are actually supporting *all* things, including ourselves. This chapter lists just a few of the ways you can give support and kindness to the world, to others, and as a result, to yourself.

I-M-U (I aM yoU)

A great way to approach giving support and kindness is to be aware of the oneness of humanity and that giving to others is giving back to you and your family. Many cultures recognized the interconnection of all things as reflected in their language. The Mayan phrase *in lak'ech ala k'in,* meaning *I am another yourself,* is used as a greeting from one human to another and shows an awareness of a person's connection not only to all humans, but to everything in existence from the smallest particle to plants and animals to the largest galaxies. The Sanskrit word *namaste* has the general meaning of *I honor the place in you that honors the place in me; we are all one.*

Many of us have experienced how great we feel when we selflessly do something for another. Perhaps the reason we feel so good is that it is true that we are all connected, like one leaf is connected to all the other isolated leaves on a tree, and that doing something for another is indeed doing something for yourself. Giving support and kindness enhances one's own health, happiness, and prosperity.

In Our Nature

When we are sufficiently nourishing our own basics of life, such as love, good food, safety, comfortable shelter, and a comfortable state of mind, it's in our nature to support and be kind to others. At the right place at the right time, most people will kindly pick up something dropped by another, help push a stuck car, open a door for someone, or smile at a stranger. Many people dream of whom they would help if they won the lottery. If we are not kind, it's not because of nature, it's because of *nurture:* think of all the city dwellers who develop street-smart attitudes to survive, or all the parents who tell their children to beware of strangers, or all those cultures and countries that hold on to resentment for hurt caused by past generations, or of the media that constantly delivers bad news into our living rooms. But at the same time, there are many "Mother Teresas" in the world. As mentioned earlier in this book, the Dalai Lama once said that there are more acts of kindness than ever before in the history of earth. We hear of individuals reaching out to depressed and suicidal souls, of rich people bequeathing their fortunes to charity, of a multitude of people just showing up to pitch in and build a house for a needy family.

Before You Give to Others, Give to Yourself

Before you give to others, it's important that you first give yourself the pledge of respect, support, kindness, and follow-through. If you have read and applied the concepts in this book, you are already well on your way to giving to your body, mind, and soul.

When you give to and respect the *I,* you can then effectively help others. For example, you could continuously give money to a relative who wastes your gift on garbage food, alcohol, drugs, or unnecessary toys. To truly help that person, you could instead show him how you gave to yourself, how you have done your work, how you recognized and controlled your own IMP and instincts, how you have controlled or completely stopped your Unhealthyolic habits, and how you have welcomed HHP into your life through your own HeLP. Only at that point can you help the other person recognize the reasons for his destructiveness and set a new path, if he so chooses.

That's the kind of help others will benefit from the most. We can still give to them as we improve ourselves, as long as at the same time we teach them to recognize their IMP and destructive instincts. And the best way to do that is to teach by example. If you see an obese, junk-food-eating, cigarette-smoking doctor or personal trainer showing other people how to care for their bodies, your inner radar tells you it doesn't make sense. For the doctor and the trainer to be most effective, they must *walk* the *talk*. The same goes for you. You have already done a great service to humanity by pledging to stop your Unhealthyolic habits.

From the place of control of your own habits and by practicing HealthyIsm, you can effectively reach out and be kind and supportive to others. Give without asking for anything in return, and you'll see that what you receive is as priceless as any piece of nature. Giving makes you feel good; it makes you feel like part of a large caring family.

Giving *Is* Receiving

One of the principles of HealthyIsm is to give a portion of the goodness that you receive in life back to the web and cycle of life. Giving out support and kindness is not a tax or an obligation, it is an opportunity to do and feel good; those who give always benefit as much as or more than those who receive.

Give to Two Others

To ensure that the practice of HealthyIsm has the support of people who have had the experience of stopping their own habits and welcoming HHP, it is important for you to give support to at least two others and do so without expecting anything in return. You can give them support in various ways: offer a listening ear, encourage them, give them a *HealthyIsm* book, teach them to *fish*, buy tools for them, or show them how you took control of your mental manipulators.

Here are some ideas for giving back to the web and cycle of

life. Remember that your acts of kindness can be spontaneous and random or planned and specific—what matters is that you practice as many as you can on a regular basis.

1. Smile at someone and say in your mind "I am another You," meaning that we are all connected. Trust me on this one—you'll likely be overwhelmed by a warm feeling, especially if the person smiles back or at least acknowledges the smile.

2. Connect to people through their eyes, looking just long enough into their eyes to show acknowledgement, admiration, unity, and respect.

3. Give to organizations that *teach people to fish* rather than those that just give people fish. Such organizations teach people to take care of themselves, to produce as much in life as they consume, or to produce more in life than they consume. Give to organizations that promote helping people find their own solutions to Unhealthyolic habits. (See HealthyIsm.com for a list of organizations that make it their mission to teach people to fish.)

4. Give this book to as many people as possible to help spread the practice of HealthyIsm. See HealthyIsm.com for greatly discounted copies of the book.

5. Volunteer at a youth center, women's shelter, or prison halfway house and offer to teach the people you meet how to control their destructive instincts and IMP.

6. Open your arms often and offer a hug; you'd be surprised how many people will accept it, even if they accept it awkwardly. You can say it's a hug for HealthyIsm!

7. Offer a listening ear to someone in need. Focus intently on what she is saying. Repeat her thoughts back a few times in your own words without offering advice or solutions. Just listen.

8. Compliment someone on something you find nice about him or her; everyone has an amazing "something," be it the eyes, voice, imagination, creativity, pleasantness, or a special talent.

9. Buy a gift of a trip to a wellness recovery retreat and offer it to someone who needs it and will commit to it, such as a homeless person, relative, or a former executive of some bankrupt mega-corporation.

10. Support the HealthyIsm Organization through a financial contribution or by helping with such aspects as administration, teaching, listening to others, and raising awareness.

11. Donate a percentage of your wealth directly to teaching others to fish.

12. Donate money to individuals or organizations that are developing cheap and clean energy sources. With all of our help, very affordable energy for all people will be a reality sooner than later.

13. Give back to someone who has helped you in the past, be it yesterday or 40 years ago. If someone has been kind and supportive to you, look into his life for a moment to see how you can help him. Call, e-mail, or send a thank-you note even for the smallest nicety. Or donate to a charity on his behalf.

14. If someone helped you as you practiced HealthyIsm and took control of your life, give back to that person in whatever way seems fit; help her plant a garden or build a house, help her children, or find a source of income or compensate her for her efforts in helping you.

Closing Thoughts

In this chaotic time of many crises and great achievement, where the decisions of today determine the future of our tomorrow, we are often reminded of Ghandi's phrase "be the change you want to see in the world." In retrospect, that is what this book is about: viewing the mending of the inner challenges of the I as the best way to support the outer challenges of the world.

This book was written not to tell people what to do, but to inspire people to welcome constructive consciousness into their lives. Most people want HHP for their children, but why not for themselves? Perhaps they *do* want HHP, but their destructive instincts and the way they have been conditioned to think get in their way. If practicing HealthyIsm (or any other method) has helped you to get out of your own way and people *ask* you how you have the ability to be in better control of your thinking, reach out and gently show them what you have done.

You often hear the line of reasoning, usually from someone trying to justify his destructive behavior, that "life is a trip and I want to finish my journey saying, 'whew, what a ride!'" To him, that means inhaling whatever, eating whatever, drinking whatever, and doing whatever his IMP and instincts want regardless of the damage it causes to his body and, by extension, to others—*and shrugging off his actions by saying they make life interesting.*

Yes, at the end of one's life there should be a "whew!" factor, but make your *ride* about being, looking, and feeling amazing! Guaranteed…that'll make life interesting. And the biggest whew! factor will be that you know in practicing a healthy *I,* you participated in passing a beautiful, healthy world on to generations to come.

Whoever you are reading this right now, I say to you: with the different abilities that you have and at your own pace, calmly and kindly look within the I of the beholder, see your own beauty, stop your Unhealthyolic behaviors, and calmly and kindly welcome a life of HHP. Thanks for playing your part in the practice of HealthyIsm! Spread the word—and if you are now in control, help at least two other people take control of their minds, too.

Namaste!

APPENDICES

Appendix A: Healthy I

Appendix B: Healthy World!

These appendices were added to offer an insight into what the author does for his own good health (touch wood!) and a foresight into what the world could look like with a society that finally wakes up and focuses on living constructively such as suggested in the practice of HealthyIsm.

APPENDIX A

Healthy I: I Am What I Do!

Calmly, and hopefully kindly, I welcome into my life the ability to stop sickness, disease, depression, and other lower levels of existence before they have a chance to develop in my body. We have something here in Canada called "Run for the Cure," an event dedicated to raising *funds* for breast cancer research, education, and awareness programs.[36] This is a great cause, and it is very much needed, but I have often thought that we must also have an event called "Run for the Optimization of Health," to raise awareness of *what we can do to help prevent all diseases in the first place*. The focus of such an event is entirely about helping and encouraging people to take the actions necessary to give their bodies the best chance of being strong and healthy. See HealthyIsm.com for information about this event.

By now we know that, even if we have the genes necessary to develop certain diseases, there are actions we can control that will highly influence whether those genes are unlocked and a disease develops or not. Two important keys to keeping those genes locked are: 1) preventing toxins and other stressors from affecting the body (such as stopping them from entering in the first place, or neutralizing their adverse effects, or moving them through and out of the body as quickly as possible); and 2) providing the body with all the movement and materials necessary to keep it optimally strong and healthy.

The main purpose of this book has been to familiarize people with and have them participate in HealthyIsm as a daily life practice. The practice includes recognizing and controlling the weaknesses of mind and, as a result, stopping Unhealthyolic habits and welcoming in sustainable health, happiness, and prosperity (HHP). Writing this book has also given me an opportunity to improve my life by practicing constructive consciousness and focusing on my *I* so that I can walk the talk and show by example.

There lies the purpose of this Appendix: to give you an idea of what I do for my health. It is a summary draft of *my walk* specifically as it relates to what I eat and how I move and exercise my body.

I am what I do…or don't do

Even though I have had my share of "downs," I still live a mostly happy and healthy life. I seldom get sick or sad, I play a lot with my children, I laugh a lot, I sing often, and I feel connected to nature and others. When asked how I do this, I say it's by being aware of the craziness of my IMP and of the weaknesses of my human nature—and by being aware that *I am what I do*.

Nutritionist Victor Lindlahr wrote a book in 1942 called *You Are What You Eat,* which suggested that food controls one's health. Today, the importance of what we eat is less of a suggestion and more of a given. With my own health, I am aware that *I am what I eat* just as much as I am what I do in many other areas of my life. For example:

- *I am* what I eat and how much I eat and what nutrients

I ultimately assimilate into my body.

- *I am* how I use my body.

- *I am* what I think.

- *I am* how my IMP controls me.

- *I am* how much I let destructive instincts control me.

- *I am* how aware I am of the world in me and around me.

- *I am* what amount of sunshine I allow to shine on me, which, among many benefits, converts to much-needed vitamin D in my body.

- *I am* what awareness (and acceptance) I have of the oneness and connectivity of all things.

- *I am* how many toxins and stressors I let affect my body or allow into my body in the first place.

- *I am* what love I give and receive.

- *I am* what joy I have and radiate.

- *I am* what relationships I have in my life.

- *I am* what resources and tools I have to support a healthy lifestyle.

- *I am* how much I play and interact with my kids.

- *I am* how much I laugh, play, sing, and dance overall.

- *I am* how much support I receive and give.

- *I am* what I do (or don't do) to my body, mind, and soul.

The state of my life and, in extension, the state of the world, is what I do in my life. Just like a musician practices his instrument every day to be his best, I practice daily doing good things (mostly as described in the HeLP of Chapter 10) for my body, mind, and soul to be my best. When I'm being calm and kind to my I, here's what I regularly do in terms of body use and nutrition:

What I Do – Body Use

Posture

I will focus on exercise in a moment, but first a little about my focus on posture for such positions as standing and bowel movements. Part of my proper use of the whole body is performing and maintaining correct posture. When walking or standing, I always stand tall as if I'm stacking my ears, shoulders, and hips in a straight line. With my hands by my side, I rotate my thumbs outwards, which forces my shoulders back and chest open. From there I practice a half-inch, navel-toward-spine squeeze and a slight buttock squeeze (as if trying to hold a coin between the cheeks). I have consciously practiced this proper posture for years, to the point where it is now a mostly unconscious behavior. It feels good and, as a by-product, looks great.

Bowel movements

I also practice proper posture for bowel movements, which means squatting on my feet on the toilet instead of sitting on my butt. A side effect of western society's inner mental programming is the unnatural position of the human body when sitting on a toilet. I'm not making this up—it's true! Like most people in western civilization, I was programmed to sit on a toilet instead of squatting my derriere right to the ground like I am naturally designed to do. Because of this, the anal tract was in a bent/kinked position, resulting in extra exertion to push feces out and therefore contributing to my development of hemorrhoids. I had heard about squatting before, but it was only about five years ago, after observing my young children naturally squatting while pooping in their diapers in the corner, that I started squatting, too, by placing my feet on the toilet seat. A little tricky, but the results were evident and motivating—my bowel movements became much easier and the hemorrhoids subsided. Yes, diet does affect the ease of evacuation, but squatting is very effective because it not only places the anal tract in the proper straight position, but it also allows the thighs to push lightly on the abdomen.[37] Okay, enough of that crap....

Just enough movement and proper use of the whole body

Too much body use wears the muscles and joints down; not enough body use makes the body weak and unhealthy. Having operated numerous injury rehab clinics, I've seen my share of manual laborers whose hands or wrists are injured from the repetitive or jarring use of a particular tool. I've seen hard-core athletes whose bodies are just broken from overuse: marathon runners with bad knees or hips; dancers with broken feet; and baseball pitchers with messed-up elbows or shoulders. Not to belittle the sacrifices of people who just want to provide for their families or are on a quest for personal excellence, but the cause of their injuries is usually wear and tear, plain and simple. The ultimate goal for me in relation to *getting the most mileage out of my vehicle* is to engage all body parts on a regular basis, but not too much. Our bodies were biologically designed to *occasionally,* over the course of a day, a week, or a season, gather food, hunt, run from being hunted, roam long distances, climb, build shelters, and so on. In doing just enough of all of these actions on a regular basis, we were able to provide all the necessities of life, which in turn had good effects on our bodies that allowed them to remain strong and healthy so they could do it all again the next time.

In knowing that, I work all of my muscles and bones at least once a week, usually twice. This means that over the course of four to five workouts per week (30–45 minutes, each workout), I make sure that I exercise all of my body parts in the many ways they were designed for or are capable of doing: pushing, pulling, lifting, squatting, walking, short bursts of running (since the body was designed for chasing prey or for running from predators), twisting, stretching, kicking, punching, throwing, catching, climbing, skipping, jumping, swimming, and so on. If I am being active, whether I'm playing a sport, engaging in vigorous gardening or intense landscaping, moving lumber and tools around while building something, hiking, playing with the kids, or exercising with clients, I will count that as a workout.

Workouts

I teach a fusion fitness class twice a week in which I fully participate. Fusion fitness means that during the course of the class, I incorporate many different fitness exercises from different disciplines, simulating the actions of various body movements used in yoga, martial arts, farming, Pilates, various sports, and traditional exercises. For example, after a good warm-up and stretch, a typical workout might look like this:

Exercises with a 15- to 20-pound weight in each hand:

- picking up a bale of hay with a proper lift, twisting, and "throwing" the bale up to the loft (20 reps in each direction)

- pause to stretch and recover

- slow motion tennis serves (20 reps each on left- and right-hand serves)

- pause to stretch and recover

- one-legged squats

- plain bicep curls, but on one foot with a slight twist

- pause to stretch and recover

Exercises with no weights:

- martial arts kicking and punching (a few intense minutes)

- five-inch push-ups (40 reps)

- pause to stretch and recover

- various yoga postures, holding position and focusing on the breathing to slow the heart rate (30–60 seconds)

- one-handed push-ups (hold each for 20 seconds, then switch hands)

- pause to stretch and recover

Continue with more exercises using weights

Then back to exercises with no weights

And so on for 25–30 minutes

Cool down:

- stretching

- yoga postures

- regeneration meditation (5–10 minutes)

The plan going into any of these fusion classes is to use the whole body in varying movements and intensities; by the time we are done we are soaked from head to toe but feeling great, feeling euphoric.

A couple of times a week I go to a local gym. When working with weights, I mix up the intensity of the workout by sometimes using extremely heavy weight and sometimes using a weight just heavy enough to do 10 reps or so. The human body has basically three different muscle fibers that are capable of a wide range of activities, from simply maintaining posture to running fast to lifting something heavy. In some workouts, I move through a wide range of motions to incorporate all muscles, and once every week or two I team up with a buddy to lift or push super-heavy weights. For sample workouts and more information on using the body, you can check out HealthyIsm.com.

What I Do – Nutrition

Just enough of the best fuels for my body

There have been 125,000 generations since the first Homo species, 7,500 generations since the emergence of the current human species, and only 500 generations since the advent of agriculture, which is regarded as the reason for the beginning of civilization.

That brings humanity's lineage to the current generation of *me*. As an observant, well-rounded human of the present civilization, I have become aware of what promotes the best health for my genetic heritage.

After years, generations, or even centuries of living a certain way or believing a certain something, it's very hard to break free, even if we know that the belief or way of living is destructive. For example, there is some evidence that eating various grains such as those normally used in bread, cereal, and pasta is harmful to some degree for most of the world population. Even though our genes and our bodies haven't had time to adapt over the brief 500 generations of mass consumption of grains, we still hold on to a belief that we must eat six to 11 servings of grains to improve or maintain our health because either Mom, the media, a dietician, or some other professional told us to do so.

My understanding, based on my studies and personal experimentation, is that I must keep grains down to a minimum, soaking or sprouting them when I do consume them, and eat a high percentage (at least 60%, and some days as high as 90 to 100%) of a raw, organic, mostly vegetable diet. I'll also have a couple of eggs (usually raw) most days and the occasional intake of meat and fish. That is when I feel my best. If I don't eat at least 60% this way, my energy and clarity diminishes and my body suffers from inflammation (especially the joints and gums). On most days, I also keep the "bad" foods to a bare minimum. I stay away as much as possible from foods that are "denatured" by harmful things like microwaving, chemicals, overcooking, and the way they were grown.

Sample of my daily intake

Remember that the information in this appendix is what works for me and may not work for everyone. I studied, experimented, listened, and experimented some more before finding out the ideal formula for myself. In fact, I am still (always) experimenting with what foods make me feel my best, but for now I am pleased with what I've come up with so far. It may sound strange, but I usually look at myself as a mostly raw-sequential-vegetarian who occasionally eats organic meat and fish (average once a week).

The first thing I do when I wake up is slowly drink a glass of clean, filtered, reverse-osmosis water from the tap mixed with a tiny pinch of Celtic sea salt. This first glass of water makes up for the water lost during sleep. About 15–30 minutes later I have a super-drink made up of a green powder mixture that contains a wide array of super-foods and that is chock-full of the vitamins, minerals, antioxidants, and enzymes that I may not find in my regular diet. I add to that a couple of tablespoons of chia seeds (yes, the same seeds used for the Chia Pet craze of the early 80s!), a tablespoon of bee pollen, and a pinch of cayenne pepper powder.

Another 30–45 minutes later, I begin to eat sequentially, which means eating one food in its entirety before moving on to the next food. I begin with sprouts, then have some type of vegetable like broccoli 15–20 minutes later, then celery, then red or yellow peppers, and so on. If I am heading out in the morning, I take some of this with me, pre-washed and ready to eat, especially the easy-to-eat foods like celery, broccoli, cauliflower, carrots, and peppers (which I eat like an apple). If I am home I usually chew and swallow a couple of raw eggs stirred in a cup (I know, yuck!). For lunch I might move away from sequential eating and have a plate with diced avocado, tomato sprinkled with olive oil and sea salt, pesto sauce, and humus. Or I might have a good-sized salad containing a mix of lettuce, avocado, kale, tomato, nuts, sesame seeds, a few raw, organic pecans, and a splash of balsamic vinegar and olive oil.

I eat two or three organic ripe fruits a day, between meals, depending on my current health condition. If I'm not feeling well, I eat very little or no fruit because the sugar in fruits may feed a disease. For snacks I eat raw organic nuts and seeds, which I soak overnight to make them easier for the body to digest. At some point during most days I use a juicer to juice a bunch of vegetables like kale, celery, red cabbage, broccoli, and lettuce, along with a piece of ginger. For supper, unless I'm taking in organic meat, or fish, I might have a hearty lentil soup poured over the leftover fiber from the juiced vegetables.

Be Practical, Not Fanatical!

I'm not fanatic about this routine (or anything else hopefully)—on occasion I do allow myself a "cheat" or unhealthy food such as an oatmeal cookie with a cup of coffee—but I do this only as a rare indulgence to bring a smile to my face, and *only* if I'm feeling great; otherwise, I avoid these cheats. I also love the taste of a glass of red wine with a meal a couple of times a week; I believe it's beneficial for me and appreciate the feeling of euphoria given by the alcohol. If I come to accept that wine causes more harm than the benefit of the phytochemicals and endorphins released into my body, or that I can't control my indulgence, I will reduce my intake or eliminate it completely from my diet.

Once every week or two, I'll have nothing during the day but freshly extracted vegetable juice (as described above) or water with squeezed lemon. A couple of times a year I go on a three- to five-day cleanse in which I drink only certain fluids and consume high-fiber agents to clean "the plumbing."

In a nutshell, here is what I currently do to ensure a healthy *I:*

1. Use my body in the ways for which it was designed in terms of posture, bowel movements, and exercises that require me to properly use all body parts in varying degrees and intensity. I do these exercises on a regular basis, but not too much.

2. Consume enough, but not too much, of a mostly sequential, raw vegetable diet with a regular or occasional sampling of nuts, meats, eggs, fruits, and sprouted or soaked grains. If feeling well, I'll eat some cooked foods and occasionally have a treat.

APPENDIX B

Healthy World!: A Story of H.O.P.E.

Feeding the body optimal nutrients and exercise helps you attain and maintain a healthy mind and body—and feeding the mind a seed of hope contributes to an optimistic outlook on life, providing perhaps a little less fear and stress in daily living. Call it daydreaming or a far-fetched imagination, but it's gratifying to think of healthy, constructive humans in a healthy, constructive world. We all have an infinite number of paths forward through our control of IMP and instincts and the choices we make. This appendix looks at welcoming a path that imagines one of many possible, optimal end states to our world's present conditions. Some of the following may seem ridiculous to you (like Galileo's heliocentric theory was?), while some may seem completely possible. As you read this story, let your imagination go wild, have fun with it, and feed the mind a seed of hope!

This is a story of H.O.P.E. (HealthyIsm Onward to a Positive Evolution), a glimpse of our Earth in the future, an Earth that has matured into a healthy, happy, and prosperous planet. Earth has survived the reckless times of its societal adolescence by humanity recognizing, controlling, and transcending the weaknesses of its instinctual nature and the destructiveness of its inner mental programming (IMP).

This story is about an alien research vessel traveling through space, time, and parallel universes on a mission to observe, connect with, research, and witness other life forms and document their findings.

In 2047, the vessel entered a milky, spiral galaxy and rapidly zoomed in on one certain star with numerous orbiting planets. From 200 million miles out, the aliens could see that the third satellite from this star was luminous, with a bluish-white glow and blots of green—the telling colors of a living planet—which they identified as Earth.

This was a planet that they had visited periodically over thousands of years, always fascinated by one of the greatest "evolutionary shows" in the universe. Each time the aliens visited, they grew increasingly interested in one of Earth's complex creatures—the one called "human." These bipeds were the dominant forms of biological life on this planet mainly because of their highly developed brains and their ability to manipulate their abundant surroundings with their limbs and hands. The aliens documented these humans on each visit, noting that they were slowly evolving entities that were still immature and inexperienced with their gifts. Humans tended to abuse their abilities and seemed to live in a persistent destructive state.

To the aliens, Earth had always been a planet worthy of ongoing observation not only for its scientific value and intriguing theatrics but also because the aliens had a vested interest in Earth's survival. They had long ago confirmed nonduality and acknowledged oneness – what was good for the humans and the earth was good for the aliens! It had been about 40 years since they last visited; they suspected that the situation could only have gotten worse.

But this time as the aliens neared the familiar planet, they noticed that something was different—the planet looked pristine and healthy. Analysis showed that the high toxic levels in the atmosphere that had been recorded during the last visit were now virtually non-existent. Other tests showed that the Earth was indeed healthy. The question was whether the destructive humans had died off, or if they had finally matured and evolved to a higher state of consciousness and overcome the weaknesses of their primal nature and thinking.

The aliens moved in closer and, following their approach protocol with their anti-detection and cloaking devices activated, selected a remote area on one of the large land masses for their exploration.

The alien ship hovered 10,000 miles above the planet, still outside its atmosphere, and transported a researcher to explore the area and, if possible, to make contact.

As the alien researcher materialized on the Earth's surface, her personal cloaking shield activated for protection, she noted her surroundings: a bluish winding river on a very lush, green landscape with a multitude of colorful plants and creatures; but no human life. After taking a few other readings and documenting her findings she began to move toward the active water. Then suddenly she stopped; she could hear an interesting sound coming from behind her; it was a human singing!

"Zip-a-dee-doo-dah, zip-a-dee-ay. My, oh my, what a wonderful day…"

She turned, and amazingly, there amidst all this beauty was

indeed a human approaching along the water bank. Had they evolved, then?

This cheerful human was Jay, a middle-aged man taking a stroll in the sun and fresh spring air. Jay was on a break from his morning chores on the organic wellness farm he and his family were visiting in central Canada.

Jay stopped suddenly; he intuitively felt something unusual in the air, but wasn't sure what it was. His first sense was a feeling of warmth and calmness.

The alien, sensing this calmness, slowly lifted her personal cloaking shield to reveal herself to this great creature.

Jay was slightly surprised, but not afraid, to see this strange, beautiful being and looked upon it with the same amount of curiosity as he would a plant or animal he'd never seen before. It had been accepted worldwide for many decades now that there were other entities in existence. He knew that ancient Earth cultures had documented in their drawings and literature the suggestion of alien encounters. And in the recent past, many people from all walks of life—including heads of state, Nobel laureates, trusted scholars, regular people, and even a few of his own friends—had described peaceful encounters with aliens. So far there had never been a report of harm or foul play. It was almost as if once a species was intelligent enough to create the power source and means to be able to travel the stars and visit other beings, wherever and however they existed, they likely had matured and evolved to a point of constructive consciousness.

The alien traveler and the earthling calmly greeted each other with eye contact, slight bows, and smiles, both subconsciously focusing on the unfolding present moment. Jay sensed that this was a kind and peaceful being. She was somewhat human-like, a little taller than Jay, who was just over six feet himself. She had long, wavy, jet-black hair, snug, dark green clothing that revealed a sculpted, strong body, brownish skin, and a culturally mixed, long smooth face with beautiful wide hazel eyes.

The being spoke briefly, her voice strange but comforting, telling Jay that she came in peace, that her name was Lamare, that she was one of the more highly evolved beings in existence, and that her ancestors had visited Earth many times before. She told him of the continued research and documentation they were doing and asked to interview him about his planet's current condition. Without hesitation, Jay agreed.

This is where we join their dialogue:

Lamare: Thank you for your calmness. Do you have an identifier?

Jay: Identifier?

Lamare: Yes. Perhaps you call it a handle, moniker...a name?

Jay: Oh, a name. Yes. Jay Deeman.

Lamare: How old are you?

Jay: Born in 1999, which makes me...47 years old.

Lamare: Please, Jay, we are interested in the last 40 years of your planet, but especially in its current state of visual beauty and intuitive calmness that we now witness. It seems obvious that something amazing has happened that has allowed you to evolve. Please tell us...

Jay thought about the request and, to refresh his memory and input data, connected telepathically to the global mental databank of information, the modern version of the archaic, original Internet (where in the old days, people had to log on, type, wait for a response, and determine what made sense). The Telepathy Internet Method, TIM, using DNA computing, began to rise in popularity around 2025 when enough humans became aware of, accepted, and were educated in its use. People had learned to tap into the conscious bank of all minds, to recognize and filter out the chatter of human minds (the IMP) and make reasonable, rational, and constructive decisions of matters of mutual importance. Through near-instantaneous collaboration of human and artificial intelligence, TIM was able to correlate and decipher all information on any subject and provide an accurate definition or answer to most questions. If not able to be answered, the question would be added to a list to be solved in queue, based on importance.

Voluntarily tuning into TIM, Jay felt honored to explain the current state of the Earth to the striking creature before him.

Jay: As you see, the world is dramatically different now in 2047 than it was not too long ago. Today it is a peaceful, healthy, happy, prosperous, and abundantly comfortable world.

Up until the first decade of the second millennium, this was a messy world filled with fear, anger, greed, scarcity, and depression, all caused by harmful belief systems that propelled issues like an energy crisis, global terrorism, human greed, national and governmental assertiveness, economical instability, and ecological destruction.

There was intense fighting locally and globally; many wars raged between nations and cultures, and regular people fought like kids bickering over a possession or a preferred seat on the school bus. Pollution was out of control. Humans held on to distrusting, hateful relationships with each other based mostly on fear and historical injustices done to and by their ancestors.

The Earth suffered from dirty air, dirty water, sick food, and the extinction of many plants and animals. The people suffered from stress, worry, and a lack of awareness of their destructive instincts and inner mental control, and they were sick and tired. The Earth was sick and tired!

Lamare: Why was it like that?

Jay: Because people didn't know any better; they were locked in the prison of their instinctual weaknesses and inner mental programming. For the longest time, whenever people were taught by their elders or institutions that something was a certain way, they believed it and would do anything, even destroy self or others, to maintain those beliefs. If a person was told that the inner walls of a house were only black, for example—and these walls were in a house the person was forbidden to enter—that person would believe it, unquestionably, without having seen the "black" walls for himself.

But then things changed…

People began to understand and use a practice called Healthy-Ism, which was all about giving oneself the best and kindest care possible in order to create a healthy self and a healthy world. In the process of creating a healthy existence people had to become aware of the control that their inner mental programming (called IMP for short) and their instincts had over them.

People began looking into the house, so to speak, and saw that the house was full of many beautiful colors.

For one thing, we saw that the Earth, as I and all humans began to accept, was like a living cell made up of many intricate elements, including its own cellular intelligence—which was partially the collective minds of humans. It became crystal clear that everything on and in Earth, all living and "non-living" matter, contributed to the cells' makeup and very existence; everything was connected and codependent in a web and cycle of life.

People everywhere recognized that everything, including humans, was part of a great unfolding sea, a universal wave of expansion and contraction of an evolutionary process. And most accepted that this process was powered by a special power, a blob of consciousness, a Universal Spirit or God, or something indescribable, which united all people together regardless of their background.

We began to understand that we were an intrinsically integrated part of this infinitely large blob of consciousness or God. Humans, having the ability to reflect on their own consciousness, could make sense of this concept by imagining themselves as a conscious point in the center of this larger blob of consciousness. We envisioned that all living and nonliving things were "in their own center" and were connected to each other and every possible thing in this blob—the past, present, future, here, there, another person, plant, animal, or distant star. We accepted that an important function of all humans within the centre of this pulsing consciousness was to be an experiencer of the larger blob self, like a baby's eyes and fingers experiences, in wonder and awe, the mystery of her own toes.

Lamare: Yes, I assumed that was the case. In my understanding it is one of the essential ingredients that helps to prevent self-destruction of any intelligent life form. Once a species realizes its role as an experiencer, they accept shared ownership of all of existence and thus more often welcome in constructive levels of consciousness. Please continue...

Jay: Thank you. Even though it looked like Earth was headed for certain destruction, it became smarter because its human mind-bank, its conscious cellular intelligence, was becoming smarter. Slowly but exponentially, as people began to be more aware of their fear-based instincts and programming and calmly question the status quo and outdated beliefs, many things began to emerge that created a more constructive society, a healthier human, and a healthier world.

We began to adapt to the changing world around us, instead of fighting change. For example, fanatic cultures and countries that held onto male-dominated mindsets began to relax and allow equality amongst all people, especially women. Another example is that, even though we continued to do everything we could to lessen our ecological footprint, we spent our energies adapting and building habitats and systems that could withstand or minimize any harshness of the changing world. We had to ride out the storm that man and nature were creating. In the process we began to live in harmony with nature. We began to walk lightly and nurture nature instead of stomping all over her.

As a society we quickly matured. We were no longer running around with an adolescent attitude of invulnerability, self-indulgence, and recklessness. Through the process of painful lessons, humans came to realize that they wanted something better. Many people, people of all nations, grew up and matured as if overnight. Basic human rights and needs were practiced and pursued first by small groups and then, exponentially, by larger groups who joined together to form a powerful, yet gentle, influential body.

Suddenly there was a global resonance of trust in the air. We knew we had to get along in this home called Earth. A peaceful consciousness began to emerge on the planet around the time of the new millennium, and we participated in global activities like worldwide grassroots meditations, international "Healthy I, Healthy World" concerts, wide-reaching webinar classes (with millions in attendance) that explored such things as how humans were unconsciously trapped in their worlds of destructive thought and instincts and therefore causing all kinds of chaos to themselves, others, and the earth.

As we woke up, the common practice was to control and stop destructive instincts, thoughts, habits, and actions, to forgive those weaknesses of self and others, and to welcome what most people wished and yearned for in their calmest and kindest state of mind, which was great health, happiness, and prosperity for self and for all.

As these practices unfolded, humans from all walks of life began asking a basic question at all times: "Is my thought or action constructive or at least neutral to self, others, or the earth?" If they answered yes, they continued on; if they answered no, then they welcomed improving that thought or action at their own pace.

Slowly, the ignorance, chaos, and fear around the world began to dissolve, and was replaced by awareness, stability, and love! Society evolved beyond the hold that outdated behaviors, beliefs, and indoctrinations had over us. As hard as it was, we changed.

For example, beginning in 2010, people everywhere followed the practice of simultaneously participating in daily breaks from their thoughts and activities to focus, meditate, or pray for at least one full minute together as a global whole. During this time, each person joined millions of others and practiced being aware of his or her own body, his or her own breath, and especially his or her own heartbeat. With this awareness of the pulse of the present moment through the heart of their bodies, people eventually learned to spread that awareness to the pulse of all things happening at that moment, including anything they could actually hear, smell, see, or feel. They also focused on the shared living earth below their feet, envisioning it and their own bodies to be healthy and vibrant. They envisioned all things, especially each human, to be connected beyond their common planet, as one within a Universal Spirit, within God, within a blob of consciousness, as if they themselves were molecules of a drop of water of one huge, infinite, and eternal ocean of oneness. Those who couldn't or wouldn't think about spirituality or oneness were encouraged to focus on something that made them calm or happy or gave them a good feeling.

Also during a focus, practitioners, either physically or mentally, placed one hand over their brain, representing control of mind, and one hand over their heart, representing acting with love.

This focus helped create a feeling of community and fellowship throughout the world. People could actually feel the resonating serenity and power created by these brief daily, global meditations.

It didn't take long for these practices to spread through the Internet and word of mouth. Before long they were picked up and practiced by cultures, countries, major religions, businesses, and other groups around the world. The practice was beautiful; it encouraged people to examine their own weaknesses first, to stop the control of any destructive instincts or IMP, and welcome in enduring happiness, optimal health, and peaceful prosperity in any kind and calm means possible.

All around the earth over the next three years, humanity constructively evolved in an exponential way never before imagined possible, and within a short time from the Mayan-prophesized judgment era of 2012, Earth's entire population was flourishing in a heaven on earth, or at least welcoming in living in peace and having great HHP. It was not the end of the physical world, as some people had feared, but the end of the destructive human mindset. It was the painful yet amazingly beautiful birthing of higher levels of human consciousness.

All people either had or were in the process of getting the basic necessities of a healthy life, like nourishing food, clean air, pure water, and safe shelter. Hospitals and schools were built and easily accessible to all people around the world. By 2020 the earth was healing nicely, destined for a full recovery but licking its scars of extinct species, devastated forests, human genocide, and other awful memories.

But awful memories did not dictate and overwhelm people's thinking. They knew better by now. They observed the memory, established the lessons, found the silver linings, forgave when necessary, and archived the recollection or memory for future personal or collective review. People knew that they were more than the negative emotions derived from any unpleasant memories.

They were now free to fill the vacuum created by releasing the heaviness of these depressing emotions with good thoughts and good feelings.

As people accepted and lived these practices, they stopped waving the errors of the past in each others' faces.

All people first focused on themselves to stop their own destructive Unhealthyolic habits that harmed themselves, others, or the earth in any way. Humans worldwide unconditionally forgave self and others for past weaknesses and craziness and habitually welcomed in optimal health, enduring happiness, and peaceful prosperity (HHP).

Lamare (recording Jay's explanation of earth's recovery): Amazing narrative; as we approached your planet we suspected that humans had either become extinct or evolved, and it's obviously the latter. What happened next?

Jay (feeling naturally high from recounting his tale): Incredible things began to unfold.

All the minds that had been giving energy to destructive forces before 2009 were now working together for the common good. Instead of giving in to unconscious, primal, protect-my-life-and-the-life-of-my-clan instincts, which we innately display as children (when we are unable to control our possessive urges of "mine, mine, mine") people were now collaborating, sharing ideas and resources, and co-creating solutions, beneficial tools, constructive services, and biologically friendly products.

Money, human manpower and *mind power,* and other resources were used to create instead of to destroy.

And boy, did humans ever co-create!

Jay transmitted this last thought to the alien with a smile, then went on.

Certain achievements in the history of humanity, like the control of fire, the invention of the wheel, the evolution of the printing press, the development of the Internet and the invention of electronic speech to speech translation of any language to *any other* language, were great gifts that allowed a little more control of one's destiny. But recognizing and controlling the destructiveness of certain instincts and one's IMP was the biggest global achievement of all time.

Through the control of our minds and cooperative constructiveness came another big achievement – the realization of low-cost, environmentally friendly, clean energy. Not only solar or wind or geothermal energy, but new technologies such as perpetual generators, crystal powers, and many other innovative, wonderful discoveries. A few people throughout history had already hypothesized about and experimented with different energy resources, but they had still been largely unknown to the masses. The only costs were for initial parts and occasional maintenance; otherwise, the various devices and units produced endless amounts of very cheap clean energy. This change revolutionized the world.

Cheap, clean energy replaced the filthy fossil fuels for all of our technology, especially transportation. We developed underground high-speed trains and reliable flying vehicles equipped with special anti-collision instruments. We were now able to carry humans and cargo, pollutant free, to all corners of the globe in a short amount of time.

We used cheap energy for heating and air conditioning. Cheap energy powered climate-controlled dwellings for growing wholesome organic plants, providing a means to nourish everyone on earth.

Oh, and the by-product of some of these *free* energy producers was water! This allowed all regions of the world access to a limitless clean water supply.

New technologies improved the lives of so many people.

Scientists, engineers and doctors worked together to create

clever diagnostic systems that were able to quickly diagnose any deficiency, illness, or diseases, allowing for corrective actions through lifestyle improvements or, if necessary, medical intervention.

But intervention was rare because people started making good lifestyle choices to begin with. They were eating well, using their bodies properly, thinking right, and living more in touch with nature.

By 2030 we collectively designed and built several massive "universe ships" commonly called "uni-ships" that held thousands of people and were capable of researching and exploring deep space and preserving human life indefinitely.

As we worked together as one, the social and ecological environment improved, and—through increased equalities and cooperation between countries, classes, individuals, and genders—peace prevailed.

We learned to give and to support and help other people and nations, expecting nothing in return, but subconsciously knowing that we would be naturally gifted in return with the peace and joy of a healthier world.

All communities worldwide were given the resources, heirloom seeds, and tools to provide healthy food, build strong, safe shelters, and develop strong, sustainable local economies.

Jay paused to take in the beauty of the moment—the fresh air, the sunshine warming his vibrant body, the sound of the babbling river, and the presence of his inquiring guest.

I would like to sit; please join me. Gestured Jay.

The alien lowered her body to a squatting position and Jay sat directly on the ground. He continued: So many other things happened…

We had the world population explosion under control by 2020; people, especially women, in all cultures were given the family planning knowledge and the materials they needed to control their own fertility, and nations kindly encouraged their citizens to limit their offspring to two or three.[38]

And amazingly, as an elective practice, most people, wealthy and poor alike, voluntarily donated 10–90% of any surplus of reserves they had toward providing the basic necessities of life for others and supporting and/or inspiring others who had had enough of their unhealthy habits and destructive ways. These donations were not handouts but a means of teaching people to "fish," to take care of the *I*. All people began to have the means to provide the basic needs for themselves and their families, and the ability to maintain such. Donations were also directed toward funding projects and jobs that created or supported constructive economies in such fields as researching and developing free energy, building comfortable, earth-friendly dwellings, growing healthy food, repairing and cleaning the earth, and helping the plants and animals.

The 20% of the world's richest population, who were consuming 80% of the world's resources, recognized that we were all part of one large family. They were now sharing what they had and investing in humanity with still plenty left over to provide a fulfilling life for their families for many generations.

As time went by, there was a leveling of resource distribution, which bettered the lives of all, with the poorest in society receiving the biggest initial benefit. People developed their talents, giving themselves the opportunity to gather resources to support basic HHP and beyond. Skilled people were paid more. Company executives were paid less but still plenty. Even though wealthier people sacrificed some of their surplus, they still had abundance and benefited tremendously from such things as a stabilization of the economy, a cleaner, healthier, and happier environment, much less crime, and a calming of the populations of the earth.

As more and more people stopped their Unhealthyolic habits and welcomed constructive consciousness, they allowed their natural talents to be developed and used in a constructive way, which gave them extra resources to welcome in even greater HHP.

Commerce also changed. It became more about sustainability and less about every man for himself. It became the blue, white, and green economy: blue for clean water, white for clean air, and green for a healthy plants and animals.. Many businesses took up these practices and eventually made all their products and services constructive, or at least neutral, to society. The world's economy was thriving and sustainable, without harming anyone!

The people began to elect blue, white, and green political parties to coach and lead, instead of govern, to lead by example and coach the team into welcoming kind and calm HHP. With coaching-style leaders we needed less bureaucracy, which in itself freed up valuable human resources.

As more people were awakened through these consciousness-raising practices, it became easier for others to awaken as well, just as it was easier mentally for those who followed in the footsteps of the first people who explored new lands, broke the speed of sound, ran a mile in under four minutes, or climbed the tallest mountains in our world. Once people recognized that many others were controlling and transcending their weaknesses and craziness, and readily welcoming in great HHP, many more followed almost naturally.

In retrospect, we realized that society had to go through the trials and tribulations of growing up in order to learn its lessons and develop the wisdom to move strongly and healthily into the future.

World peace became a reality. Humans recognized that all turmoil, conflicts, retaliation, reckless deeds, and "evil deeds" were issues that needed to be resolved and put to rest. Much turmoil was steadily resolved using non-violent techniques like focusing on and improving the *I* of each individual by being aware of destructive instincts and inner mental programming. With this awareness, long-standing conflicts were put to rest through collective evaluations and worldwide votes via the Internet.

In hardened grievances where one side appealed the collective solution, representatives of each conflicting party lived together for a short period of time, consuming healthy foods, meditating, and attending seminars on conflict resolution and the practice of constructive living.

Mutual decisions were made. People focused on the future benefits of a resolution, not the damages of the past.

Instead of handing out excessive punishments like lengthy prison sentences or execution, we started sending people convicted of crimes to "courage camps" where they received transformational caring therapies. One such therapy was nutritional healing, which got rid of toxins in the inmates' bodies and provided them with substantial nutrients and a base for healthy bodies and, most importantly, healthy minds.

With a more compassionate, healthy society, offenders also had the opportunity to be listened to, to be understood, to tell their stories about how they arrived at this point in their lives. From there, inmates were taught to recognize their lack of control over instinct and IMP—and the system worked; the rate of recidivism dropped to almost nothing. Most crimes were the result of the ignorance, recklessness, and immaturity of the individual and of society. Society up until this point had been competing within a scarcity mindset. But once people recognized this, things changed. The mindset changed to abundance for all, and cooperation. Yes, some people remained locked up for a long period of time, but they were accepted as they were, forgiven for their weaknesses and acts of craziness, and treated as part of the great oneness. Even these people were able to be productive and contribute to society by such things as raising organic gardens and giving input to the collective mind.

There was local joy and global harmony in the air, a constant feeling of being *in the zone*.

As people became aware of their weaknesses and began to control or stop their Unhealthyolic habits, they became healthier, developed stronger immune systems, and needed fewer drugs and vaccines for their disappearing diseases, maladies, and toxic mindset. It became clear to the majority exactly what was necessary to attain and maintain great health, including consuming proper foods, exercising, having ample amounts of sunshine, and taking in much-needed supplements such as vitamin D3 when lacking direct sunshine to the body.

Most children labeled as hyperactive or problematic, who were in the past medicated or institutionalized, were now recognized as victims of outdated harmful belief systems, unhealthy foods and lifestyles, or just having a different energy level, and when treated properly returned to a healthy, constructive, and joyful nature.

Even pharmaceutical companies became aware of their IMP and harmful instincts and began to improve their ways; they began to use the monies they had made off a sick, immature, and "fix my symptom of disease model" society to diversify into wellness-supporting constructive services and products. The health of all people, inspired by the executives' very own children, became the "bottom line." The new accounting spreadsheet became all about how many lives they helped to restore and maintain optimal health with natural products and services. Yes, medications were still necessary for various situations and diseases but by and large most conditions were prevented by optimizing nutritional and lifestyle choices.

We recognized that most babies of every culture and region, until they were taught otherwise, were the same loving, playful, and inquiring beings. All children were equally accepted as special because of their hope, freshness, high energy, and innocence, and they began to have a collective say in how the world evolved. Virtual classes were set up that welcomed children from all nations and religions and other possible labels, where children were taught all things in an unbiased format while welcoming in a *yes* to the basic question. These children, who represented the diverse yet unified world, became key solution makers of the future.

All plants and animals became respected by most people. The whole earth moved toward a largely vegetarian organic diet of at least 50% raw vegetables. Those people who occasionally ate animal protein to optimize health did so without gluttony or disrespect; people became conscious of their eating. No animal or plant died in vain to feed humans. Each human recognized the sacrifice of a plant or animal, that he or she would assimilate the goodness of the nutrients into all parts of the body. As they ate slowly and consciously and in small but sufficient quantities, people verbally or mentally pledged to the food in front of them that they would live in a way that was constructive, or at least neutral, to self, others, and the world.

Excessive consumption and fanaticism was replaced with moderation.

Religions were recognized beyond any inherent, obvious, or hidden destructive weaknesses as a guide for society at large to live together spiritually as one, in complete cooperation. People of all denominations broke through any "my way or the *hell way*" roadblocks ingrained in their IMPs, acknowledged the similarities between each other's religions, and began to cooperate despite historical differences or interpretations.

All religious and spiritual groups united together in "spirit-tanks" to brainstorm and work together to understand the essence of each other's beliefs and of life, and how they could get along together once and for all. Religious or atheist or something in between, it didn't matter; we all began to work together in harmony. Instead of developing weapons of mass destruction, we developed tools of mass construction.

Lamare: Can you give an example?

Jay: Sure. We realized that there are many possible *unfoldings* of our future, and the global tribe chose what we have today. In 2034, humans collectively worked together to develop a strategy to divert a large asteroid that was certain to strike the earth. The asteroid would have surely destroyed most life on the planet.

The alien, who looked like an innocently curious, happy, and wide-eyed child, transmitted the thought: Please, share a little more of your story.

Jay continued his telepathic dialogue: With pleasure.

If people needed support, support was there. If a person or even a nation was lacking the basics and had poor resources, mechanisms were set in place to help them.

There were challenges in the first few years: only a trickle of the world's population started living and being constructive—but soon enough there was a steady flow until the dam of unawareness and destructive living broke open to a flood of awareness and constructive living.

Aggressive, destructive people or groups who stubbornly refused to change, to do the "constructive thing," threatened to destroy the world if they didn't get their way. But as they began to witness an increasingly changing, evolving, more compassionate world, the aggressive ones' demands began to change into declarations like, "I am awake and aware…there is a better way…I will start with me." The collective, all of earth, was able to send a message loud and clear to these confused souls: "We are all connected; each of us is like a blade of grass connected on the great lawn of humanity. We are in control of the weaknesses of our nature and our minds, not the other way around."

The aggressive ones began to recognize their own weaknesses and reach out for help, to create health, happiness, and peaceful prosperity for themselves and for their nations. As a result the world needed less police, less border security, and less military. Borders still exist today as a means to preserve the positive aspects of cultural identity and to protect people from those who occasionally get lost in the destructive aspects of their IMP and instincts.

Lamare at this point was radiating a beautiful transparent golden aura. She looked at Jay and grinned: What you humans have achieved is out of this world.

Jay: There is more, but of the same…shall I go on?

Lamare slowly rose to her feet: I have heard enough, and I am a witness to the truth that you speak, to the reality of the beauty you and your kind have evolved into and have created for the inhabitants of this planet.

We, like many other entities that we've encountered in our travels, went through similar challenges as we matured as a species over eons of time, and we eventually controlled our thoughts and instincts and developed into the peaceful participants and observers of the evolutionary process that we are today. We've come to know and accept that our general purpose, as it is for all existence, is to calmly and kindly participate in and be witness to all that is, to Universal Spirit/God's self.

I will say this: we are pleased that you have adapted and evolved with the practice of constructive consciousness. It is of benefit not only to your planet and its inhabitants, but to all existence, because just as you have realized that you are all connected on Earth, you are also connected to me. Your evolution is our evolution. Healthy human, healthy *I!*

Jay, sensing that this encounter was almost over, stood up, smiled, and held open his arms as an offer of peace and love. The alien recognized the universal sign, leaned over, and embraced Jay for a brief moment that seemed timeless. She then stepped away from Jay, smiled slightly, and said,

May optimal health, enduring happiness, and peaceful prosperity always be with you.

And also with you, *whispered Jay* …until next time..

Lamare slowly dematerialized and transported to her waiting vessel to continue on her journey. Jay stood for a second, basking in the warm, mixed sensations of awe, joy, love, and sunshine. As he mused over his brief close encounter, he found himself quietly humming "Zip-a-dee-doo-dah…". He then turned and strolled back to the wellness retreat to share his experience and story of H.O.P.E.

The end?

Notes and Resources

1. Barbara Marx Hubbard, producer and narrator, Humanity Ascending, Prod. Quantum Productions, DVD. In association with The Foundation for Conscious Evolution.

2. Dr. Joseph Mercola, "Are You Sabotaging Your Plan to Exercise?" October 30, 2008, http://articles.mercola.com/sites/articles/archive/2008/10/30/are-you-sabotaging-your-plan-to-exercise.aspx (accessed December 12, 2008).

3. David R. Hawkins, Power vs. Force: The Hidden Determinants of Human Behavior, 1 ed. Sedona, AZ: Veritas Publishing, 1995.

4. "Quantum Computing," July 22, 2008, IT Acumens, http://discuss.itacumens.com/index.php?topic=17551.0 (accessed July 14, 2008).

5. Wikipedia contributors, "The Journey of Man: A Genetic Odyssey," Wikipedia, The Free Encyclopedia, http://en.wikipedia.org/w/index.php?title=The_Journey_of_Man:_A_Genetic_Odyssey&oldid=282117093 (accessed July 14, 2008).

6. Wikipedia contributors, "Galileo Galilei," Wikipedia, The Free Encyclopedia, http://en.wikipedia.org/w/index.php?title=Galileo_Galilei &oldid=294169393 (accessed July 23, 2008).

7. Wikipedia contributors, "Milgram experiment," Wiki-

pedia, The Free Encyclopedia, http://en.wikipedia.org/w/index.php?title=Milgram _experiment &oldid=293471308 (accessed May 31, 2009).

8. Joseph Chilton Pearce, Magical Child. New York: Plume, 1992.

9. Ronnie Falcao, LM MS, Licensed Midwife, "Umbilical Cord Issues," GentleBirth, http://www.gentlebirth.org/archives/cordIssues.html# Delayed (accessed August 2, 2008). This article lists several other resources pertaining to umbilical cord and home birth issues.

10. Swami Jnaneshvara Bharati, "Training the Ten Senses or Indriyas," http://www.swamij.com/indriyas.htm (accessed June 12, 2008).

11. Wikipedia contributors, "Intuition (knowledge)," Wikipedia, The Free Encyclopedia, http://en.wikipedia.org/w/index.php?title=Intuition_(knowledge)&oldid=293886899 (accessed May 2, 2008).

12. Liz Kimmerly, "Love Is the Answer," June 2008, Divine Caroline, http://www.divinecaroline.com/22108/51608-love-answer/2 (accessed August 2, 2008).

13. John Dewey, "The School and the Life of the Child," Chapter 2 in The School and Society, Chicago: University of Chicago Press, 1907; 47-73.

14. Stambor, Zak, "Bonding over others' business," Monitor On Psychology. 2006;37(4):58. http://www.apa.org/monitor/apr06/bonding.html (accessed June 2, 2009).

15. Allen Carr, The Easy Way to Stop Smoking: Join the Millions Who Have Become Non-Smokers Using Allen Carr's Easyway Method, 1 ed. New York: Sterling, 2005.

16. Wikipedia contributors, "Rat Park," Wikipedia, The Free Encyclopedia, http://en.wikipedia.org/w/index.php?title=Rat_Park &oldid=278962221 (accessed September 17, 2008).

17. "Saturated Fats Good?" February 12, 2008, B Welling, http://bwelling.wordpress.com/2008/02/12/saturated-fats-good/ (accessed September 23, 2008).

18. Mike Geary, "Is Saturated Fat Evil, or Not So Bad After All? The myths, lies, and misconceptions about saturated fat and your health," Truth About Abs, http://www.truthaboutabs.com/saturated-fat-is-not-evil.html (accessed September 23, 2008).

19. Wikipedia contributors, "Soloman Asch," Wikipedia, The Free Encyclopedia, http://en.wikipedia.org/w/index.php?title=Solomon_Asch&oldid=291104129 (accessed May 22, 2008).

20. Wikipedia contributors, "Victor Lebow," Wikipedia, The Free Encyclopedia, http://en.wikipedia.org/w/index.php?title=Victor_Lebow&oldid=294251326 (accessed June 3, 2008).

21. Eckhart Tolle, A New Earth: Awakening to Your Life's Purpose. New York: Dutton, 2005.

22. Hopi Elder (unnamed), "A Hopi Elder Speaks," Hopi Nation, Oraibi, AZ, http://www.communityworks.info/hopi.htm (accessed July 6, 2009).

23. David R. Hawkins, "The Map of the Consciousness" in Power vs. Force: The Hidden Determinants of Human Behavior, 1 ed. Sedona, AZ: Veritas Publishing, 1995.

24. Deb Gebeke, "Children and Fear," April 1994, North Dakota State University, http://www.ag.ndsu.edu/pubs/yf/famsci/he458w.htm (accessed October 24, 2008).

25. Andrew Cohen, "OpEd," EnlightenNext Magazine. 2009;43:14.

26. Inspired by an August 2008 seminar conducted by Paul Chek. For more information about Paul and the C.H.E.K. Institute, visit http://www.HealthyIsm.com.

27. Stanley S. Bass, "Super Nutrition and Superior Health," Life Science International Fasting Center, http://www.drbass.com/freedownload/files/drbassdotcom3.pdf (accessed November 2, 2008).

28. Inspired by the writings of Barbara Marx Hubbard, Humanity Ascending; Andrew Cohen, EnlightenNext Magazine; and Steve Pavlina, StevePavlina.com.

29. Influenced by the writings and teachings of Byron Katie and Bruce Greyson.

30. Wikipedia contributors, "Pierre Teilhard de Chardin," Wikipedia, The Free Encyclopedia, http://en.wikipedia.org/w/index.php?title=Pierre_Teilhard_de_Chardin&oldid=292380379 (accessed May 26, 2008).

31. BBC News, "Organic Food 'Better' for Heart," July 5,

2007, http://news.bbc.co.uk/go/pr/fr/-/2/hi/health/6272634.stm (accessed January 18, 2009).

32. Influenced by the work of Dr. Karim Dhanani of the Centre for Biological Medicine. For more information on his work and the Centre, visit the website at http://www.biologicalmedicine.com/index.html.

33. Byron Katie, "The Work," http://www.thework.com/thework.asp (accessed June 25, 2008).

34. Eckhart Tolle, A New Earth: Awakening to Your Life's Purpose; 191.

35. Rabbi Chaim Kramer and Rebbe Nachman of Breslov, Anatomy of the Soul, 1 ed. Jerusalem: Breslov Research Institute, 1998; 364.

36. For more information about this important event, visit the Canadian Breast Cancer Foundation's Run for the Cure website at https://www.cibcrunforthecure.com.

37. Stephanie Relfe, "Squat, Don't Sit! Change your toilet so you can heal constipation (and many other health problems)," Health, Wealth & Happiness, http://www.relfe.com/toilet_seat_constipation.html (accessed May 18, 2009).

38. Eddie Rose, "The World Population Explosion," July 6, 1998, Yale-New Haven Teachers Institute, http://www.yale.edu/ynhti/curriculum/units/1998/7/98.07.06.x.html (accessed May 30, 2009).

ABOUT THE AUTHOR

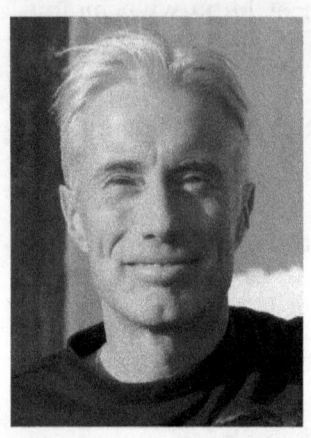

Gary Drisdelle has studied extensively in the fields of wellness, fitness, addiction, life coaching, motivation, and nutrition and has supported hundreds of people in their quests to welcome more constructive lives. He considers that most people are inherently good; that humanity, over thousands of years, has been "growing up"; that humans as a collective have barely survived the irresponsible stage of our adolescence; and that we are destined to exponentially mature into the next stage of an optimally healthier, enduringly happier, and peacefully prosperous condition. Gary is based near Toronto, Canada.

Give to Two Others

If you found that this book has helped you in some way you may be thinking of how you can let others know about it. Here are a few ways:

Give to two others. One of the principles described in the practice of constructive consciousness is to lock in what you have learned by showing at least two others how you have changed. Think about the people in your life who are a bit (or a lot) lost in their own destructive habits. Calmly and kindly give this book as a gift without expecting anything in return.

Reach out to the media and let them know about the book and how it has changed your life. Call, write or email your local newspaper, radio and television stations and suggest that they contact the author through the HealthyIsm website.

Let all the people in your life know about HeatlhyIsm through word of mouth, your email lists, social networking sites and so on. Talk about this book on your website or blog. Tell them the story of how it has helped you or how you have witnesses others change as a result of practicing the principles in the book.

Books are available at substantial discounts when used to support others in practicing constructive consciousness. Gift a set of books to various organizations, shelters, prisons, rehab centres and so forth where people may benefit.

For updated ideas, additional copies, and discount information visit *www.HealthyIsm.com*. Thank you!

www.ingramcontent.com/pod-product-compliance
Lightning Source LLC
Chambersburg PA
CBHW020741160426
43192CB00006B/235